EMERGING APPROACHES IN NOVEL DRUG DELIVERY SYSTEM

EMERGING APPROACHES IN NOVEL DRUG DELIVERY SYSTEM

Dr. Preeti Singh
Dr. Gunjan Singh
Prof. (Dr.) Amrish Chandra
Dr. Nayyar Parvez

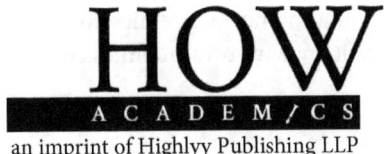

an imprint of Highlyy Publishing LLP

ISBN: 978-93-6009-172-9 (Hardback)
First Published : 2024
Copyright ©Author

Publisher's Note:

All Rights reserved under International Copyright Conventions. No part of this publication may be reproduced, stored in a retrieval system, or transmitted in any form or by any means, electronic, mechanical, photocopying, recording or otherwise without the prior written consent of the publisher and the copyright owner.

The content of this book is the sole expression and opinion of its author(s), and not of the publisher. The publisher in no manner is liable for any opinion or views expressed by the author(s). While best efforts have been made in preparing the book, the publisher makes no representations or warranties of any kind and assumes no liabilities of any kind with respect to the accuracy or completeness of the content and specifically disclaims any implied warranties of merchantability or fitness of use of a particular purpose.

The publisher believes that the contents of this book do not violate any existing copyright/intellectual property of others in any manner whatsoever. However, in case any source has not been duly attributed; the publisher may be notified in writing for necessary action.

Published by :

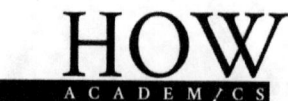

Correspondence
Address :

an imprint of Highlyy Publishing LLP
4/30 A II Floor, Double Storey Buildings
Vijay Nagar, Delhi-110009
Editorial: +91 9811026449
Sales : +91 9999953412
Email: info@howacademics.com
Website: www.howacademics.com

Contents

Preface ix
Acknowledgment xi

1. **Controlled Drug Delivery Systems** — 1
   - Introduction — 2
   - Terminology or Definition of Control release Dosage forms — 2
   - Biopharmaceutic and Pharmacokinetic aspects in the design of Controlled Release Oral Drug Delivery Systems — 6
   - Desired Biopharmaceutic Characteristics of Drug to Qualify for Cdds — 7
   - Mechanistic Aspects for Oral Controlled release Drug Delivery Formulation — 10
   - Classification of Controlled Release System — 15
   - Factors Influencing the Design and Act of Controlled Release Products — 17

2. **Polymers** — 21
   - Polymer used in Control Drug Delivery System — 21
   - Polymers as Biomaterials for Delivery-Systems — 21

3. **Micro Encapsulation** — 27

4. **Mucosal Drug Delivery system** — 35
   - Formulation considerations of buccal delivery systems — 38
   - Mechanism of buccal absorption — 43

5. **Transdermal Drug Delivery Systems** — 47
   - Introduction — 47
   - Anatomy of Skin — 49
   - Chemical Enhancers — 54
   - Physical Enhancers — 55
   - Formulation Approaches of TDDS — 58

6. **Gastro-retentive Drug Delivery System** — 63
   - Introduction — 63
   - Application of GRDDS — 70

7. Naso-Pulmonary Drug Delivery System — 73
- Introduction — 73
- Factors Influencing Nasal Drug Absorption — 75
- Nasal Sprays — 76
- Pulmonary Routes of Drug Delivery — 78
- Formulation of Pressurized Metered Dose Inhalers — 82
- Nebulizers — 83

8. Implantable Drug Delivery Systems — 87
- Introduction — 87
- Concept of implants — 88

9. Targeted Drug Delivery — 91
- Introduction — 91
- Strategies of Drug Targeting — 93
- Carriers for Targeting Drugs Liposomes — 96
- Classification — 97
- Monoclonal Antibodies — 104

10. Ocular Drug Delivery System — 109
- Introduction — 109
- Drug delivery systems to anterior segment of the eye — 114
- Drug delivery systems to posterior segment of the eye — 120
- Advanced delivery system — 121
- Vesicular system — 124

11. Intrauterine Drug Delivery System — 127
- Introduction to Intrauterine Drug Delivery System — 127
- Anatomy and Physiology of the Female Reproductive System — 129
- Types of Intrauterine Drug Delivery Systems — 132
- Design and Development of Intrauterine Drug Delivery Systems — 134
- Pharmacokinetics and Pharmacodynamics of Intrauterine Drug Delivery — 136
- Conclusion and Summary — 143

12. Principles of Drug Delivery — 149
- Drug Absorption, Distribution, Metabolism, and Excretion (ADME) — 149
- Introduction to Absorption — 151

	↳	Distribution	153
	↳	Excretion	157
	↳	Pharmacokinetics and Pharmacodynamics	160
	↳	Drug Release Mechanisms	162
13.	**Emerging Trends and Technologies in Novel Drug Delivery Systems**		**169**
	↳	Advanced Biomaterials and Polymers in Drug Delivery	173
	↳	Gene and Cell Therapy Delivery	178
14.	**Protein and Peptide Drug Delivery Systems**		**185**
	↳	Physicochemical Properties of Proteins and Peptides	186
	↳	Delivery Routes and Administration Strategies	188
	↳	Formulation Approaches for Protein and Peptide Delivery	190
	↳	Stability and Preservation of Protein and Peptide Drugs	192
	↳	Enhancing Drug Delivery Across Biological Barriers	194
	↳	Applications of Protein Peptide Drug Delivery Systems	198
	↳	Future Perspectives and Emerging Technologies	200
	↳	Conclusion and Summary	201

Glossary   **207**
Index   **209**

Preface

In the dynamic landscape of pharmaceutical sciences, the field of drug delivery stands at the forefront of innovation, constantly evolving to meet the challenges posed by diverse therapeutic needs. As we navigate the intricate realm of drug delivery, the quest for more efficient, targeted, and patient-friendly approaches has given rise to a plethora of emerging strategies. This book, titled "Emerging Approaches in Novel Drug Delivery Systems," encapsulates the cutting-edge advancements and novel paradigms that researchers, scientists, and practitioners are exploring to revolutionize drug delivery.

The journey into the pages of this book unveils a tapestry of ingenious solutions and inventive methodologies designed to enhance drug efficacy, minimize side effects, and optimize therapeutic outcomes. From nanotechnology-based platforms and biomaterials to advanced formulation techniques, each chapter delves into a distinct facet of drug delivery, providing a comprehensive overview of the latest breakthroughs in the field.

Through the collective wisdom of esteemed contributors, this compilation serves as a valuable resource for academics, researchers, and industry professionals seeking to stay abreast of the most recent developments in drug delivery systems. The chapters not only elucidate the principles and mechanisms behind these emerging approaches but also offer insights into their potential applications across various therapeutic areas.

As we stand on the cusp of a new era in pharmaceutical sciences, this book serves as a beacon guiding us through the uncharted waters of innovation. The amalgamation of scientific rigor, technological prowess, and a vision for improved patient care resonates throughout these pages, inspiring a shared commitment to advancing the frontiers of drug delivery.

May this compilation serve as a catalyst for further exploration, collaboration, and breakthroughs, fostering a collective journey towards a future where drug delivery systems not only address current challenges but also pave the way for unprecedented therapeutic possibilities.

Acknowledgment

The completion of this book, "Emerging Approaches in Novel Drug Delivery Systems," represents the culmination of collaborative efforts and the generous support of Prof. (Dr.) Amrish Chandra Dean School of Pharmacy and Dr. Nayyar Parvez, Gunjan Singh, Sharda University. We extend our heartfelt gratitude to all those who contributed to the realization of this endeavor. I want to sincerely thanks Mr. Himanshu Singh for his inspiration, guidance and support, I also wish to note my gratitude to my husband Himanshu Singh for his effort to helping in editing of this book.

First and foremost, we express our sincere appreciation to the authors who dedicated their time, expertise, and passion to craft insightful chapters that form the core of this book. Your commitment to advancing the field of drug delivery has enriched the content.

We would like to acknowledge the reviewers whose constructive feedback and meticulous evaluations have played a pivotal role in maintaining the academic rigor and quality of the chapters. Your dedication to ensuring the scholarly integrity of this work has been invaluable.

Our appreciation extends to the editorial and production teams whose meticulous efforts transformed the manuscript into its final published form. Your professionalism, attention to detail, and commitment to excellence are evident in every page of this book. We are greatful to the academic and research institutions that provided a conducive environment for the authors to conduct their research and contribute to the knowledge presented in this volume. Thank you to everyone who played a role, big or small, in making this book a reality.

Chapter 1
Controlled Drug Delivery Systems

The appearance of oral sustained therapy forms in the 40s & early 50s drove the research into controlled-release systems as a new study field. At the outset, in the 1970s, the process of release of fertilizer and of marine anti foulants in the 1950s came into surgical practice only for one particular purpose in pharmacology. Pharmacology and pharmacokinetics have illuminated and ultimately proved the imperativeness of the rate of medication delivery for precise clinical intervention. The overall objective in such circumstances is the development of release control. Brand name of the controlled release drug is the new kind of drug formulation. At approximately 900 A.D., Rhozes introduces, or invents, the art of creating pills whose coating is mucilaginous. After this process was extensively applied by different European nations in the 10th century, several drugs, such as pearl-coated medications and tablets whose coating consists of silver and gold, came into existence with the objective of slowing or speeding invention of useable tablet coatings around that time, like enteric and drug coating. Sometime in the period 1938 to late 30s, with the coming of a new coating, second drug was codified and added to sugar coating on the tablets. This was the initial enteric coating of tablets.

Regardless, this ethnopharmacist was the first person to obtain a patent on a sustained oral release preparation; he developed a miniature coated bead that released the drug gradually and constantly. Subsequently, with the introduction of the controlled release concept Blythe was the first pharmaceutical company manufacturing a controlled release medication in 1952. During the last thirty years, the treatment of the drug delivery systems sector has been evolving because of the implementation of effective marketing strategy. Moreover, CRDDS recognition as the most appropriate approach in pharmaceutical industry that is widely adopted by many drug manufactures today. Currently, this technique along with oral as an approach for flying fans of narrow-based medicines, which have a low biological half-life and high solubility ability for water, is one of the most used methods. Besides oral administration, there are other drug delivery methods i.e. transdermal, ophthalmic, vaginal, and parenteral strains to achieve controlled drug release.

Three eras comprise the history of controlled release technology. 1950–1970 was the time frame for sustained drug release was involved in determining the requirements for the control of drug delivery from 1970 to 1990. The controlled release technology period of post-1990.

Introduction

Optimal usage of the medicine in issue, fewer doses required, maintaining drug levels within a particular range, and improved patient compliance are all possible outcomes of controlled drug delivery systems. Even though these benefits might be substantial, it is also important to consider the potential drawbacks, which include the potential toxicity or non-biocompatibility of the materials used, undesired degradation byproducts, the necessity of surgery to implement or remove the device, the patients' occasional discomforts from the delivery application, and the higher cost of using the controlled delivery form over compared to regular types of medications. As far as a perfect controlled delivery system is concerned, it should be administration and removal friendly, compatible with the physiology, mechanically strong, inert, comfortable to the patient in his/her body and should not release unintentionally, as well as be easily constructed and sterilized. Getting these points to produce a high blood level of the medication for a prolonged period of time is what many of the first controlled release devices Conventional medications delivery options, include getting blood level after medication dosage to then fall until next one. The most important face of classic drug administration is maintaining the concentration of the drug in the blood between a minimum value -that is when the drug action efficiency drops shown- and a maximum value connected to the signs of overdose toxicity.

Terminology or Definition of Control release Dosage forms

"The one for which the drug release characteristics of time course and/or location are chosen to accomplish therapeutic or convenience objectives not offered by conventional dosage forms such as solutions, ointments, or promptly dissolving dosage forms" is how the United States Pharmacopoeia (USP) defines1 the modified-release (MR) dosage form. An extended-release (ER) dosage form is one type of magnetic resonance (MR) dosage form. It is one that, when compared to a conventional dosage form (a solution or a prompt drug-releasing dosage form), permits at least a two-fold reduction in dosing frequency or a notable increase in patient compliance or therapeutic performance. The terms "extended release" have also been used interchangeably with "controlled release (CR), prolonged release, sustained or slow release (SR), and long-acting (LA)."

Controlled Drug Delivery Systems

A controlled drug delivery system distributes the medication either locally or systemically at a predetermined pace for a predetermined amount of time. Extended Pharmacological Release. With sustained release, a certain medication can be delivered at a predetermined rate and for an extended amount of time. Products with a prolonged release system gradually release the active components and last longer.

A dosage of a medication is administered over a longer period of time by a prolonged-release drug. Sustained release or prolonged release systems do not qualify as controlled release systems since they only maintain therapeutic blood or tissue levels of the drug for a longer amount of time. They differ from rate-controlled drug delivery systems, which rely on straightforward in vitro testing to precisely determine the release rate and duration in vivo. The distinction between sustained release and controlled release, Controlled drug delivery is the administration of the medication for a predetermined amount of time at a predetermined pace. Perfect zero order release, or the drug's release throughout time regardless of concentration, is known as controlled release. A sustain release dosage form is one in which part of the drug, or the initial dose, is released immediately to produce the desired therapeutic response more quickly. The remaining portion, or the maintenance dose, is then released gradually to produce a therapeutic level that is prolonged but not maintained constant. Sustained release refers to the drug's gradual release over an extended period of time. It might or might not be released under control.

Drug targeting, on the other hand, has the ability to control the spatial release of a drug within the body, making it a type of controlled release.

Rationale

The fundamental idea behind a controlled release drug delivery system is to maximize a drug's utility by minimizing side effects and curing or controlling a disease condition as quickly as possible with the least amount of drug administered via the most appropriate route. This is achieved by optimizing the drug's biopharmaceutics, pharmacokinetics, and pharmacodynamics properties. Certain aspects, such as dosage management, regulated release rate, and site targeting, are absent from the immediate release drug delivery method. Over the course of a prescribed treatment period, the drug should be delivered via an optimal drug delivery system at a rate determined by the body's needs.

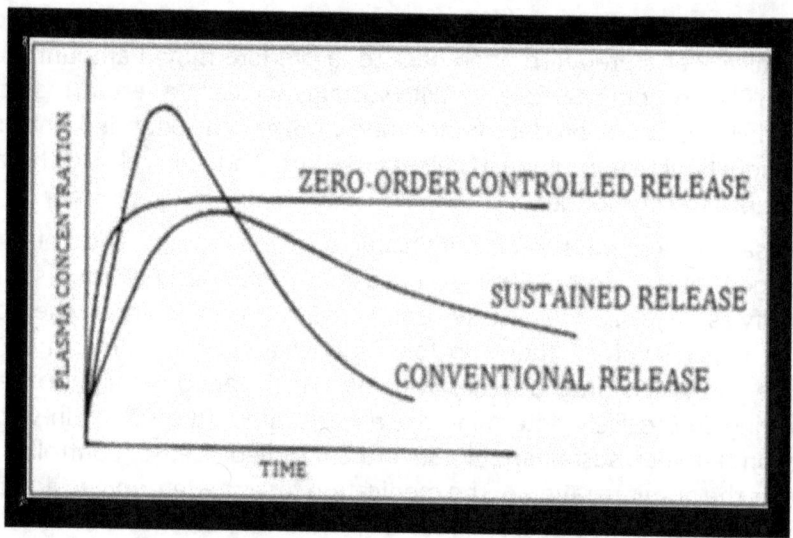

Fig.1-Plasma drug concentration- Time profile

Advantages of Control Release Dosage Forms Clinical Advantages

- Decrease in the frequency of medication administration
- Increased adherence from patients
- Minimization of blood drug level fluctuations
- Lower overall drug use in comparison to traditional therapy
- Decrease in medication accumulation with long-term treatment
- Diminished systemic/local medication toxicity
- Medical condition stabilization (due to more consistent drug levels)
- Enhancement in the bio availability of certain medications due to spatial regulation
- Economical for both the patient and the healthcare providers

Commercial/Industrial Advantages

- A demonstration of technology and innovative leadership
- Product life-cycle extension
- Product differentiation
- Market expansion
- Patent extension

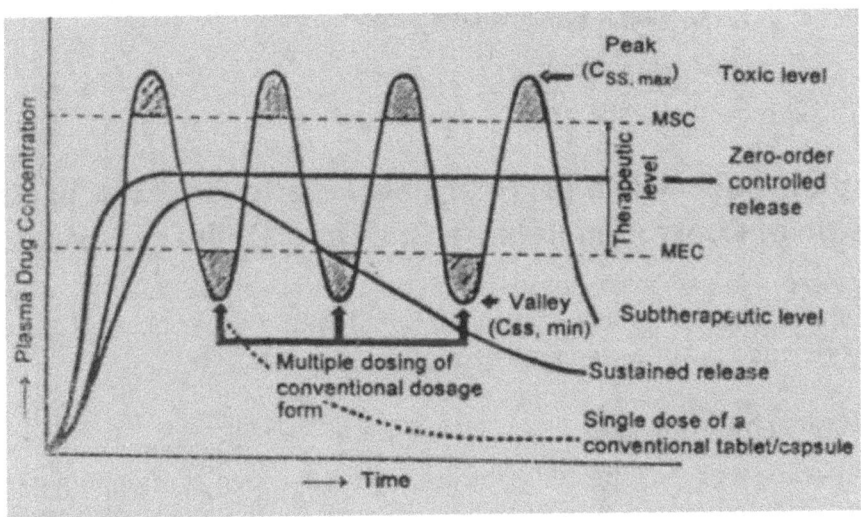

Disadvantages of CRDDS

- Delayed onset of medication effect
- Potential for dosage dumping in the event of an inadequate formulation plan
- Enhanced capacity for first-pass metabolism
- A stronger reliance on the dose form's GI residence time
- Potential for less precise dosage modification in specific situations
- Compared to normal doses, the cost per unit dose is higher
- Not every medication can be formulated into an extended-release dose form.

The most important stage is choosing the medicine to be formulated into an extended release dosage form. The options listed below are typically not appropriate for ER dosage forms.

Selection of drug candidates or characteristics that may make a drug unsuitable for Control release dosage form

- Short elimination half-life
- Long elimination half-life
- Narrow therapeutic index
- Poor absorption

- Active absorption
- Lowor slow absorption
- Extensive first pass effect

Biopharmaceutic and Pharmacokinetic aspects in the design of Controlled Release Oral Drug Delivery Systems

Drugs are released from dosage forms in controlled release drug delivery systems at a predetermined rate that is based on the drug's pharmacokinetic properties and the intended therapeutic concentration.

Biological half-life (t½)

When a drug is dosed repeatedly, the oscillations between its maximum steady state concentration and its maximum steady state concentration will be greater the shorter its t½. Therefore, it is necessary to administer medication products more regularly.

Minimum effective concentration (MEC)

If a minimum effective concentration, or MEC, is needed, one of two options is available: either a controlled release preparation or frequent dosage of a traditional medicinal product.

Dose size and Extent of duration

The delivery system's overall dose per unit must be larger the longer the time. The amount of medication that can thus be added to such a system is virtually limited.

Relatively long t1/2 or fluctuation desired at steady state

For medications with a half-life of 12 hours or longer, some people think that neither an SR nor a CRDDS are necessary or helpful. This is untrue, as there appear to be two instances where a 12 or 24 CRDDS is necessary:

1. Every two to three days, a medicine with a t ½ between 12 and 72 hours may be intended for a CRDDS allowing application. The drug's t ½ will determine how quickly the blood level time curve declines once the drug is released from the body. As a result, there may naturally be a sizable variation between Css max and Css min; in other words, this adds a delayed release to the slow elimination process. Some medications with t1/2 values between 20 and 100 hours may be more suited for

long-term usage if there are little swings between peaks and troughs at constant states because to the limited therapeutic spectrum or to attain a specific therapeutic effect.

Desired Biopharmaceutic Characteristics of Drug to Qualify for Cdds

Molecular weight or size

Convective transport is a mechanism by which small molecules can move through membrane holes. This holds true for both the passage of the drug over a biologic membrane and its release from the dosage form. The limit for biologic membranes could be 400 kcal for chain-like substances and 150 kcal for spherical molecules.

Solubility

The drug must be present in solution form at the site of absorption for all modes of absorption to occur. Determining the drug's solubility at different pH values is essential for the Preformulation study. In an acidic solution, a solubility of less than 0.1 µg/ml may result in variable and reduced bioavailability. Absorption and availability are likely to become reduced by dissolution if the solubility is less than 0.01 µg/ml. Thus, the diffusion's driving power might not be sufficient. When taken orally, it appears that medications are well absorbed by passive diffusion from the small intestine if at least 0.1 to 1% are in non-ionized form.

Apparent partition coefficient (APC)

APC requirements for drugs that are absorbed via passive diffusion must be met. In an n-octanol/buffer environment, the flow across a membrane for many medicines increases with increasing APC. The GI tract's whole pH range should have the APC determined. In order to divide the medication between CRDDS and the biological fluid, the APC must also be applied.

General absorption mechanism

A medication must absorb through diffusion over the whole gastrointestinal system in order to be a variable candidate for per oral CRDDS. In this context, "diffusion" refers to the two possible absorption pathways: entering the lipid membrane and traveling through water-filled channels between the cells. Furthermore, it is crucial that absorption takes place from all GI tract segments. This can be contingent on a number of factors, including the drug's pKa, the segment's pH, the drug's affinity for mucus, blood flow rate, etc. The GI lumen's hydrodynamics appear to have a significant impact on the absorption process.

Although zero order release profile is thought to be the ultimate ideal, first order and square root of time release can produce very effective drug delivery systems. Only two conditions must be met for zero order release in vitro release to result in zero order in vivo release and absorption:

1. The GI tract as a whole must behave as a single compartment model, meaning that the various segments are homogeneous with regard to absorption.
2. The drug release rate must be the rate-limiting step in the absorption process.

Conversely, as time increases with first order release, progressively fewer units are released per unit of time. Relative to the small intestine, less medication is absorbed if the rate of absorption slows down because of greater viscosity, less mixing and less intestinal surface area. Enzymes in the lumen, peristalsis, pH variations in the GI tract, etc. should not, in any scenario, affect the drug release from the CRDDS. A CRDDS for the majority of medications can be designed effectively using the one compartment open paradigm, in all actuality.

Pharmacokinetic parameters Elimination half life (t½)

CRDDS is best suited for drugs with a half-life of eight hours. The dose amount that must be included in a dosage form with a 12- or 24-hour duration may be too large if the t ½ is less than one hour. A CRDDS is typically not necessary if the t ½ is particularly long, unless the goal is to only lessen the variability of steady state blood levels.

Totalclearance (CL)

The volume of drug distribution cleared in a certain amount of time is measured by CL. It is the crucial factor in determining the steady state concentration and the necessary dose rate for CRDDS.

Terminal disposition rate constant (Keorλz)

The elimination rate constant, also known as the terminal disposition rate constant, can be derived from the t ½ and is necessary for forecasting a blood level time profile.

Apparent volume of distribution(Vz)

The volume that a drug would presumably fill (Vz) if it were dissolved at a concentration equivalent to that of blood. It is the proportionality constant that

Controlled Drug Delivery Systems

connects the body's total drug content to the blood's measured concentration. The first two parameters in the trio CL, Vz, and t ½ are the independent variables, and the final parameter is the dependent variable. To forecast the concentration time profile, one has to know the Vz or CL.

Absolute bioavailability (F)

The percentage of a medicine that enters the bloodstream after being administered extravascularly is known as its absolute bioavailability. One desires a F value that is near to 100% for medications that are appropriate for CRDDS.

Intrinsic absorption rate constant (Ka)

For a drug supplied orally as a solution, the intrinsic absorption rate constant must be high—generally an order of magnitude higher than the targeted release rate constant of the drug from the dosage form—to ensure that the release mechanism is the one increasing the rate.

Therapeutic concentration (Css)

The target or desired steady state minimal concentrations (Css min), the mean steady state concentration (Css avg), and the desired or target steady state peak concentrations (Css max) are the therapeutic concentrations. The variation is the difference between Css max and Css min. The accuracy of the dosage form performance must be higher for smaller desired fluctuations. Less medication needs to be added to a CRDDS; the lower Css, the smaller Vz, the longer t ½, the higher F, and so on.

Approaches to design controlled release formulations

1. Dissolution controlled release
   - Encapsulation Dissolution control
   - Seed or granule coated
   - Microencapsulation
   - Matrix Dissolution control
2. Diffusion controlled release
   - Reservoir type devices
   - Matrix type devices
3. Diffusion and Dissolution controlled systems
4. Ion exchange resins
5. Osmotically controlled release

Mechanistic Aspects for Oral Controlled release Drug Delivery Formulation

Dissolution controlled release

A solid material that has been dissolved in a particular solvent is called dissolution. This phase determines the rate at which liquid diffuses from solid. Several theories explain dissolution:

Diffusion layer theory, Surface renewal theory, Limited salvation theory.

Noyes Whitney Equation $dc/dt = kD.A(C_s-C) dc/dt = D/hA.(C_s-C)$

dc/dt = Dissolution rate,

k = Dissolution rate constant (1st order),

D = Diffusion coefficient/diffusivity,

C_s = Saturation/maximum drug solubility,

C = Conc. Of drug in bulk solution,

C_s-C = concentration gradient,

h = Thickness of diffusion layer.

Two common formulation systems rely on dissolution to determine release rate of drugs are:

Encapsulated dissolution system

Matrix dissolution system

Encapsulated dissolution system

The term "Coating dissolution controlled system" is another name for this. The stability and thickness of the coating determine the pace of coat dissolution. It reduces GI discomfort and hides flavor, odor, and color. Drugs that are highly water soluble can be made into controlled release products by slowing down their rate of dissolution. This can be achieved by making the right salt or derivatives, covering the drug with a substance that dissolves slowly, or integrating the drug into a carrier that dissolves slowly. Examples are Chlortrime to Repetabs and Ornade spansules.

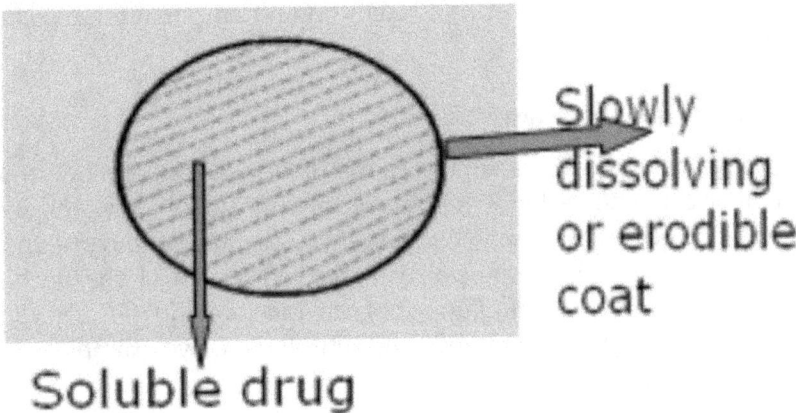

Soluble drug

Matrix dissolution system

Martrix dissolution controlled system is another name for it. This dissolution can be regulated by changing the tablet's porosity, making it less wet, or dissolving more slowly. It comes after medication release in first order. The pace at which the polymer dissolves can be used to calculate the medication release. Dimetapp extentabs and Demeaned extencaps are two examples.

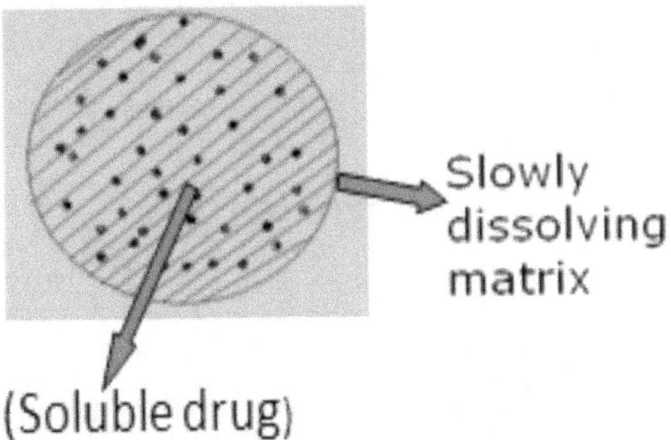

(Soluble drug)

Diffusion controlled system

It is a significant absorption mechanism that requires no energy. This drug's diffusion, which is directly proportional to the concentration gradient across the membrane, occurs when molecules move from an area of greater concentration to one of lower concentration until equilibrium is reached. Diffusion of the release rate through a water insoluble polymer governs this system. There are two varieties of diffusion devices: matrix diffusion system and reservoir diffusion system.

Reservoir diffusion system

An alternative name for it is a laminated matrix device. It's a hollow structure with an inner core encased in a membrane that is insoluble in water, and the polymer can be added by coating or microencapsulating. Drug partition into a membrane and exchange via diffusion with the fluid around it is the mechanism that controls the rate of the drug. Epoxy, polyvinyl acetate, and HPC are examples of frequently used polymers. Nico-400 and Nitro-Bid are two examples.

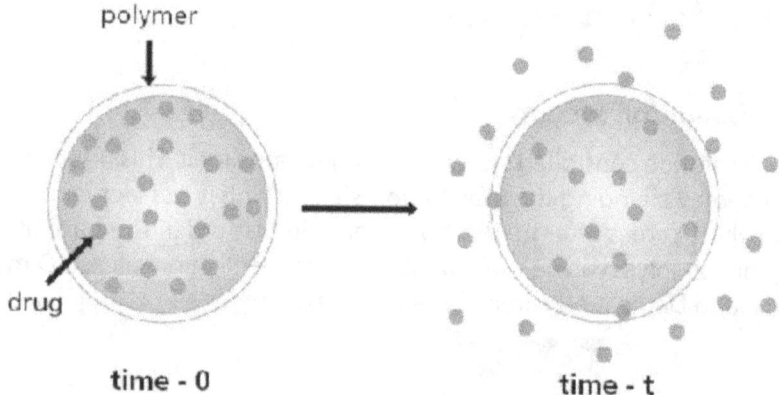

Rate controlling steps: Polymeric content in coating, thickness of coating, hardness of microcapsule.

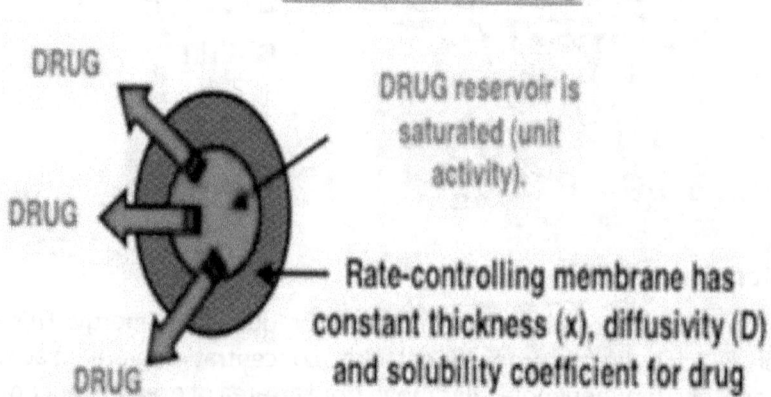

Reservoir Drug Delivery System

Matrix dissolution system

The matrix erosion systems are the most frequently encountered techniques for modulation of the input, and it brings about the uniform distribution of active pharmaceutical ingredients throughout the polymer matrix. The degrading of the polymer (sometimes emanating by erosive mechanism) subsequently deliver an effective drug to its surrounding.

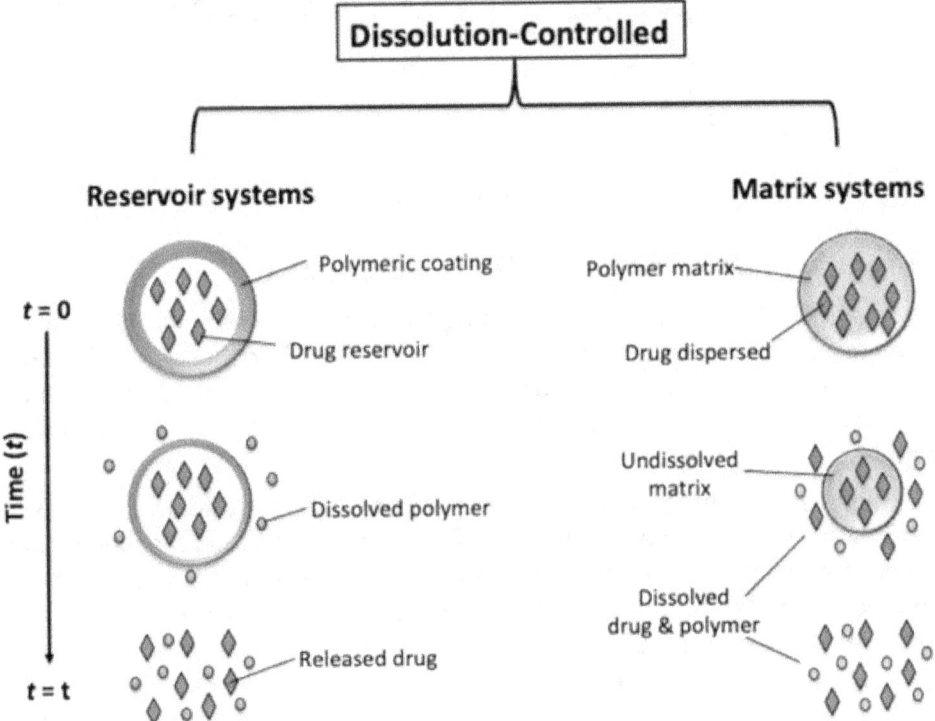

Dissolution Controlled System Flow Chart

Matrix Monolith Drug Delivery System

Either the active drug as a solution or as a matrix, the molecules are dissolved or dispersed ina matrix. In contrast to the membrane of the reservoir system, that is, the matrix system is not buried in a limiting membrane in a rate limiting membrane. Accordingly the drug release from the matrix-based structure often not be anticipated to have constant release and rather slow down the process over time.

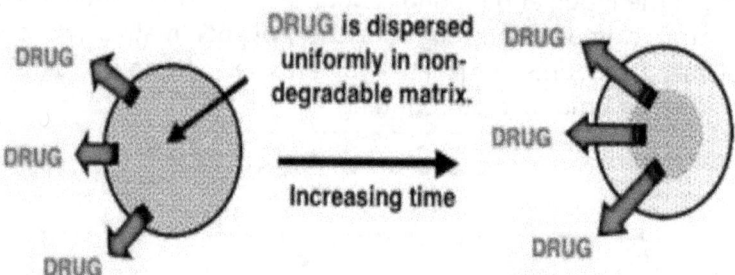

Matrix Monolith Drug Delivery System

Dissolution &Diffusion Controlled Release system

As a result of the soluble nature of coating film seems to offer a way that makes water to get inside and accompanied by dissolution of drug that occurs through diffusion of the released drug out of the system. The combined drug carrier of water-soluble PVP and water-insoluble ethyl cellulose is what makes this happens.

This medication has a membrane that is only partially soluble, and as a result, some of the membrane dissolves, leaving pores. It allows the medication to dissolve or diffuse out of the system and allows aqueous medium to enter the core. For example, the mixture of ethyl cellulose and PVP dissolves in water and forms insoluble ethyl cellulose pores.

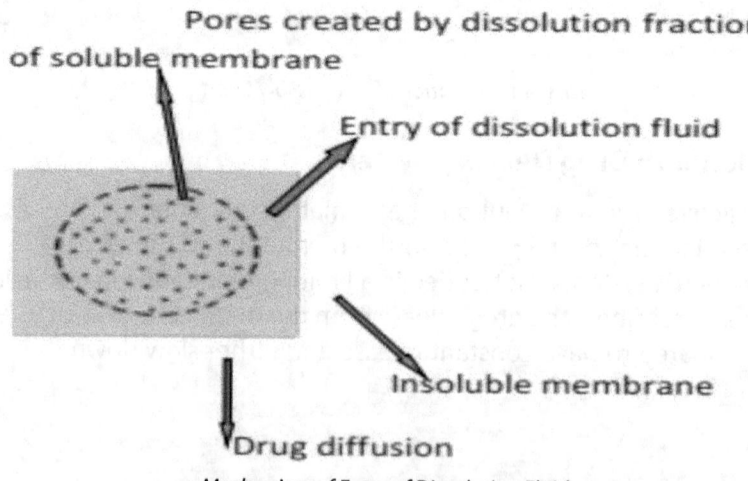

Mechanism of Entry of Dissolution Fluid

Ion exchange resins controlled release system

Water-insoluble polymers with cross-links that include ionizable functional groups are known as ion exchange resins. These resins are employed in controlled release systems and flavor masking. The drug molecules are incorporated into the ion-exchange resin matrix to create the formulations, and this core is subsequently covered in a semi-permeable coating substance such ethylene cellulose. System slowed down the medication's breakdown in the GIT. Di-vinyl benzene sulphonate is the most often used and secure ion-exchange resin available. Ion-exchange resins have been employed as a disintegrant in tablet formulations.

Table 1: Marketed drug products with their mechanism based classification

S.No.	Technology		Brand name	Drug	Manufacturer
1.	Diffusion controlled system		Welbutrin XL	Bupropion	GlaxoSmithKline
2.	Matrix system tablet		Ambien CR	Zolpidem tartarate	Sanofi-Aventis
3.	Method using ion exchange resin		Tussionex Pennkinetics ER suspension	Hydrocodon Polistirex and Chlorpheneramine Polistirex	UCB Inc.
4.	Methods using osmotic pressure	Elementary osmotic pump	Efidac 24@	Chlorpheneramine Maleate	Novartis
		Push-pull osmotic system	Glucotrol XL@	Glipizide	Pfizer Inc.
5.	pH independent formulation		Inderal@ LA	Propranolol HCL	Wyeth Inc.
6.	Altered density formulation		Modapar	Levodopa and Benserazide	Roche Products, USA

Classification of Controlled Release System

The controlled release system divided in to following major classes based on release pattern.

1. Rate pre-programmed drug delivery system
2. Activated modulated drug delivery system
3. Feedback regulated drug delivery system
4. Site targeting drug delivery system

Rate pre-programmed drug delivery system:

This involves a specific medicine flow rate profile that is pre-planned for the release of the drug molecule from the delivery device. The drug molecules' molecular diffusion within or outside of the delivery system's barrier medium is regulated by the system.

Polymer membrane permeation controlled system

This device encapsulates the drug either fully or partially within a drug reservoir cubicle. A polymeric membrane that controls flow rate covers the drug-releasing surface of the cubicle. A solid drug, a dispersion of solid drug particles, or a concentrated drug solution in a liquid or solid type dispersion media can all be found in a drug reservoir. The polymeric membrane can be synthesized as a partially microporous, semipermeable, homogeneous, or heterogeneous non-porous membrane.

Polymer matrix diffusion-controlled system

The drug's reservoir is created by uniformly spreading the drug particles within a hydrophilic or lipophilic polymer matrix at a rate that is controlled. The medicated disk has a specified thickness and a defined surface area thanks to the resulting medicated polymer matrix.

Micro-reservoir partition controlled system

The drug reservoirs consist of a solid particle suspension in an aqueous solution of a polymer that is miscible with water. High dispersion techniques are used to prepare the micro-dispersion partition controlled system. Briefly put, micro-reservoirs are created via matrix dispersion and reservoir.

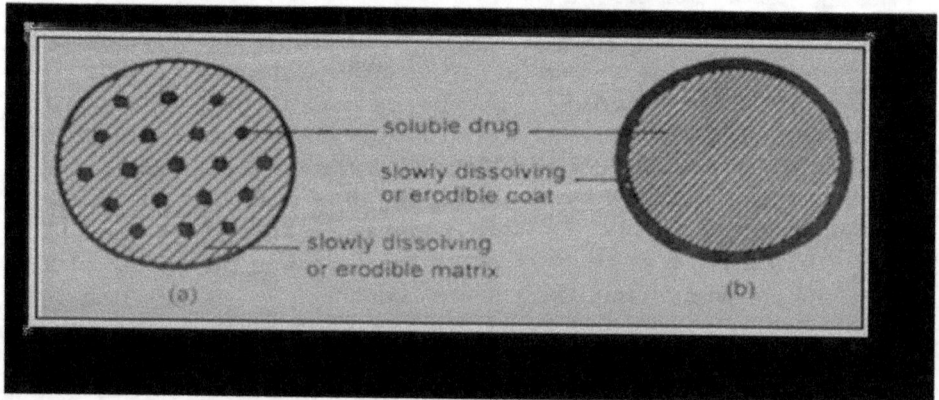

Matrix and membrane type delivery systems

Factors Influencing the Design and Act of Controlled Release Products

Physiological Properties

1. **Aqueous Solubility's**: The majority of the active pharmaceutical component (API) has weakly basic or acidic properties, which have an impact on the API's water solubility. It is challenging to create controlled release formulations for weakly water soluble medications. Drugs with high water solubility exhibit burst release and a sharp rise in plasma drug concentration. These kinds of medications are suitable candidates for CRDDS. Moreover, the pH-dependent solubility makes CRDDS formulation difficult. Drugs classified as BCS class III and IV are not good candidates for these kinds of formulations.

2. **Partition coefficient (P-value):** P-value indicates the drug's proportion in the oil and aqueous phases, which has a major impact on how the drug diffuses passively through biological membranes. Drugs with high or low P values shouldn't be used in combination with radiation therapy; they should dissolve in both stages.

3. **Drug pKa:** The drug's ionization in the GIT at physiological pH was determined by pKa. Drugs with significant ionization are typically not good choices for CRDDS. Compared to ionized medicines, unionized pharmaceuticals are rapidly absorbed through biological membranes. The range of pKa for an acidic medicine, whose ionization is dependent on pH, is 3.0 to 7.5, while the range for a basic drug is 7 to 11.

4. **Drug stability:** Medications that exhibit stability in stomach fluids, enzymatic breakdown, and acid/base conditions are suitable candidates for CRDDS. Drugs that break down in the stomach and small intestine are not good candidates for controlled release formulations since the drug's bioavailability would be reduced.

5. **Molecular size & molecular weight :** Two significant variables that influence a molecule's diffusibility across a biological membrane are its size and weight. Drug diffusion is hampered by molecules larger than 400D, although smaller molecules diffuse more readily.

6. **Protein binding:** The drug-protein combination serves as the drug's plasma reservoir. Because protein binding lengthens the biological half-life, drugs with significant plasma protein binding are not ideal candidates for CRDDS. Therefore, continuing the medication release is not necessary.

Biological Factors

1. **Absorption:** An essential component in creating the CRDDS is uniformity in the rate and degree of absorption. The drug's released dose form is the rate-limiting stage, though. To avoid dose dumping, the rate of absorption should be faster than the rate of release. The several elements that impact medication absorption include water solubility, log P, and acid hydrolysis.

2. **Biological half-life (t1/2):** The medication generally requires regular doses due to its short half-life, making it an excellent option for a controlled release device. Long half-lives of drugs necessitated dosage after extended periods of time. Drugs with half-lives of two to three hours are ideally good candidates for CRDDS. We do not use drugs with t1/2 longer than 7-8 hours in controlled release systems.

3. **Dose size:** The CRDDS must have a higher dose than a standard dosage form because it was created to eliminate recurrent dosing. However, the dose utilized in the traditional dosage form provides a guideline for the dosage needed in the CRDDS. As long as the continuous dosage volume meets the acceptance criteria, it should be as high as possible.

4. **Therapeutic window: For** CRDDS, medications having a limited therapeutic index are not appropriate. The delivery mechanism would result in dose dumping and eventual toxicity if it was unable to regulate release.

5. **Absorption window:** Drugs that exhibit absorption from a particular GIT segment are not good candidates for CRDDS. Medications that are well absorbed in the GIT are suitable for controlled release.

6. **Patient physiology:** The patient's physiological state, including factors like residential time, gastric emptying rate, and GI disorders, can have a direct or indirect impact on the drug's release from the dose form.

Controlled Drug Delivery Systems

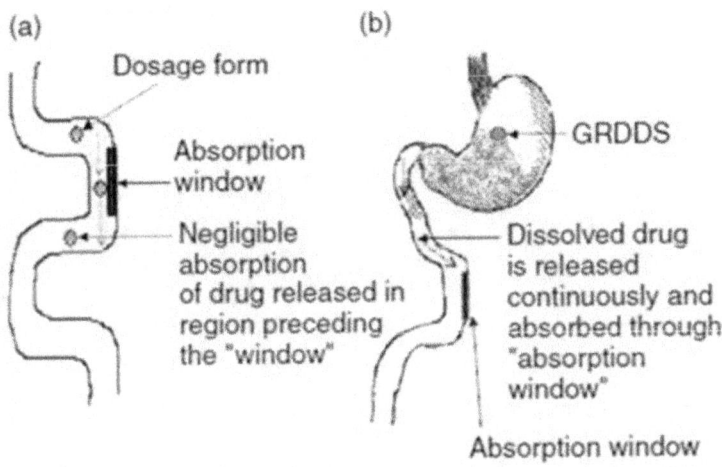

Absorption window

Pharmacokinetic parameters consider during the drug selection listed as follow:

Parameter	Comment
Biological or elimination half-life	Should bebetween 2 to 6hrs
Elimination rate constant(KE)	Required for design
Total clearance (CLT)	dose independent
Intrinsic absorption rate	should be greater than the release rate
Apparent volume of distribution (Vd)	Vd effect the required a mount of the drug
Absolute bio availability	Shouldbe 75% or more
Steady state concentration(Css)	lower Css and smaller Vd
Toxic concentration	The therapeutic window should be broader

Chapter 2
Polymers

Polymer used in Control Drug Delivery System

Drug delivery is a subject in which polymers are playing a bigger role. Polymers find usage in pharmacological applications as viscosity and flow regulating agents in liquids, suspensions, and emulsions, as well as binders in tablets. Drugs can have their bad taste covered up, their stability improved, and their release characteristics changed by using polymers as film coatings. For applications involving controlled drug distribution, the paper primarily discusses the importance of pharmaceutical polymers. With the help of sophisticated drug delivery systems, 60 million people today are able to get safer and more effective dosages of the medications they require to treat a range of illnesses, including cancer. Controlled Drug Delivery (or CDD) is the process of carefully combining a medication or other active agent with a polymer—natural or synthetic—so that the active ingredient is released from the material according to a predetermined schedule. For an extended duration, the release of the active agent can be either continuous or cyclic, or it can be initiated by external events or the surrounding environment. Regardless, the goal of regulating drug distribution is to create more efficacious therapies while removing the possibility of both under- and overdose.

Polymers as Biomaterials for Delivery-Systems

To regulate the release of medications and other active agents, a variety of materials have been used. The first of these polymers were chosen due to their favorable physical qualities and were initially meant for other, non biological purposes, such as: Poly(urethanes)for elasticity.

- Poly(siloxanes)or silicones for insulating ability.
- Poly (methylmethacrylate) for physical strength and transparency.
- Poly (vinylalcohol) for hydrophilicity and strength.
- Poly (ethylene) for toughness and lack of swelling.
- Poly (vinyl pyrrolidone)for suspension capabilities.

A material needs to be chemically inert and devoid of leachable contaminants in order to be employed successfully in controlled drug delivery formulations. It must also be easily processed, have a suitable physical structure, and exhibit less undesirable aging. Presently, a few of the materials being utilized for controlled medication delivery include

- Poly(2-hydroxyethylmethacrylate)
- Poly (N-vinyl pyrrolidone).
- Poly(methyl methacrylate).
- Poly(vinyl alcohol).
- Poly (acrylic acid).
- Polyacrylamide.
- Poly (ethylene-co-vinyl acetate).
- Poly (ethyl eneglycol).
- Poly (methacryli cacid).

Polymers:-

- Insoluble, inert-polyethylene, polyvinyl chloride, methyl acrilate, ethylcellulose.
- Insoluble, erodible–carnaubawax, stearyl alcohol, castor wax.
- Hydrophilic–methyl cellulose, hydroxyl ethyl cellulose, sodium carboxy methyl cellulose, sodium alginate.

In a matrix system, a water-insoluble polymer, like polyvinyl chloride, forms a porous matrix in which the medication is distributed as a solid particle.

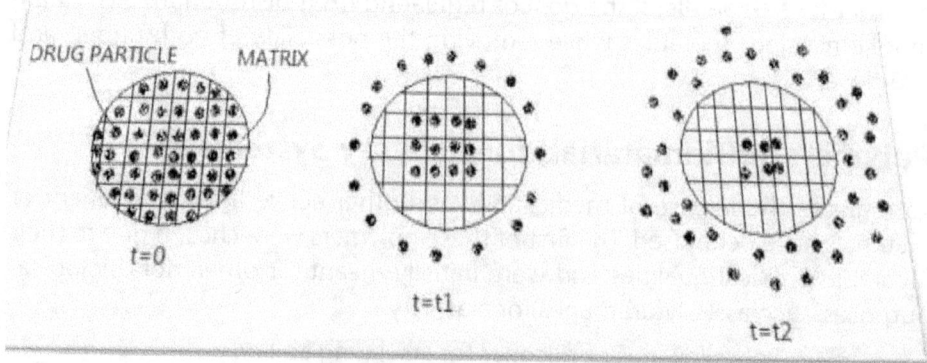

Drug Particle Matrix (t=0, t=t1, t=t2)

The drug will be released quickly after the drug particle on the release unit's surface dissolves. Following that, drug particles that are progressively farther away from the release unit's surface will dissolve and be released by diffusion via the pores to the outside of the release unit. The amount of drug in the matrix, the porosity of the release unit, and the drug's solubility are the primary formulation factors that allow the release rate from matrix systems to be regulated.

Nonetheless, more polymers with a focus on medicine have entered the controlled release market in recent years. A few of the materials among the many that are intended to break down inside the body are as follows:

- Polylactides (PLA).
- Polyglycolides (PGA).
- Poly(lactide-co-glycolides)(PLGA).
- Polyanhydrides.
- Polyorthoesters.

It was only logical to use polylactides and polyglycolides in controlled drug delivery systems as they were first employed as absorbable suture material. These biodegradable polymers' main benefit is that they disintegrate into molecules that the body can process and eliminate through regular metabolic processes. Nonetheless, biodegradable materials do release breakdown byproducts that need to be accepted by the biological environment with little to no negative effects. There are several variables that will impact how the original materials biodegrade, therefore these degradation products—both desired and possibly undesirable—need to be thoroughly evaluated. The following is a list of the numerous significant variables that show the range of structural, chemical, and processing characteristics that can influence biodegradable drug delivery systems:

- Chemical structure
- Chemical composition
- Distribution of repeat units in timers
- Presence of ionic groups
- Presence of unexpected units or chain defects.
- Configuration structure.
- Molecular weight.
- Molecular-weight distribution.
- Morphology (amorphous/semi crystalline, micro structures, residual stresses).

- Presence of low-molecular-weight compounds.
- Processing conditions.
- Annealing.
- Sterilization process.
- Storage history.
- Shape.
- Site of implantation.
- Adsorbed and absorbed compounds (water,lipids,ions,etc.).
- Physico chemical factors (ion exchange, ionic strength,pH).

References

Allen LV, Popvich GN, Ansel HC. Ansel's Pharmaceutical dosage form and drug deliverysystem.8th ed. 2004;260-263.

Bechgaard H, Nielson GH. Controlled release multiple units and single unit dosage. Drug Dev. and Ind. Pharm. 1978;4:53-67.dx.doi.org/10.3109/03639047809055639

Brahmankar DM, Jaiswal SB. Bio pharmaceutics and Pharma cokinetics: Pharmacokinetics. 2nd ed. Vallabh Prakashan,Delhi:2009;399-401.

Gibaldi M. Bio pharmaceutics and clinical pharma cokinetics. 3rd ed. Philadelphia: Lea & Febiger;1984.

Gupta S, Singh RP, Sharma R, Kalyanwat R, Lokwani P. Osmotic pumps: A review. Int.journalofcomprehensivepharmacy.2011;6:1-8.

Handbook of pharmaceutical controlled release technology. Marcel Dekker Inc. 2000;1-30.

Jain NK. Controlled and novel drug delivery.CBS publisher and distribution.1997;1-25.

John C, Morten C, The Science of Dosage Form Design, Aulton: Modified release peroraldosageforms.2nded.ChurchillLivingstone.2002;290-300.

Kamboj S, Gupta GD. Matrix Tablets: An important tool for oral controlled release dosage form. Pharma info. Net.2009;7:1-9.

Kar RK, Mohapatra S, Barik BB. Design and characterization of controlled release matrix tablets of Zidovudin. Asian J Pharm CliRes.2009;2:54-6

Lachaman L, LibermanHA, Kanig JL. The theory and practice of industrial pharmacy. 3rded.Bombay:Varghesepublishinghouse1987.

LeeVHL. Controlled Drug Delivery Fundamentals and Applications: Influence of drugpropertieson design.2nded. Marcel Dekker, Inc. NewYork: 1987;16-25.

Mamidala R, Ramana V, Lingam M, GannuR, Rao MY. Review article factors influencing the design and performance of oral sustained/controlled release dosage form. Int.journal of pharmaceutical science and nanotechnology.2009;2:583.

Modi Kushal, Modi Monali, Mishra Durgavati, Panchal Mittal, Sorathiya Umesh, Shelat Pragna. Oral controlled release drug delivery system: An overview. Int. Res. J. Pharm. 2013;4(3):70-76.

PatrickJS.Martin'sPhysicalPharmacyandPharmaceuticalSciences.3rded. VarghesePublishingHouse.Bombay:1991;512-519.

RobinsonJR,LeeVH.Controlleddrugdelivery.2nded.MarcelDekker,1987;4-15.

TripathiKD. Essentials of Medical pharmacology. 5thed.NewDelhi: Jaypee Brothers Medical Publishers(P)Ltd; 2003.

Venkata raman DSN, Chester A, Kliener L.Anover view of controlled release system.

VyasSP,KharRK.Controlleddrugdelivery:ConceptsandAdvances.1sted. Vallabhprakashan;2002; 156-189.

Wise DL. Handbook of pharmaceutical controlled release technology.Marcel Dekker Inc. NewYork: 2002;432-460.

Y.W. Chien. Novel drug delivery system.Volume50.

Chapter 3
Micro Encapsulation

The technique of enclosing or wrapping solids, liquids, or even gasses within a second material with a continuous covering of polymeric materials that produces microscopic particles (varying in size from less than 1 micron to several hundred microns) is known as microencapsulation. Thin coating is applied to small discrete solid particles or small liquid droplets and dispersions in this method to preserve the environment and regulate the availability or release properties of coated active substances. The procedure of microencapsulation is commonly used to alter and postpone the release of drugs from various pharmaceutical dosage forms. The elements that are enclosed or enveloped within the microcapsules are referred to as the nucleus, core materials, or payload materials, while the materials that surround them are called wall materials or coating materials.

Microparticles:
"Microparticles" refers to the particles having the diameter range of 1 to 1000μm, irrespective of the precise exterior and/or interior structures.

Microspheres:
"Microspheres" particularly refers to the spherically shaped microparticles within the broad category of micro particles.

Microcapsules:
"Microcapsules" refers to microparticles with a solid, liquid, or even gaseous center encircled by a coat or wall material(s) that differs noticeably from the core, payload, or nucleus.

Micro capsules can be classified on three types(**Fig.1**):
1. **Mononuclear**: Containing the shell around the core.
2. **Polynuclear**: Having many coresen closed within shell.
3. **Matrix type**: Distributed homogeneously in to the shell material.

Classification of Microcapsules

⇩ Mononuclear   ⇩ Polynuclear   ⇩ Matrix type

Fig: Classification of microcapsules

Advantages of microencapsulation:
1. Shielding the encased active agents or core components from the environment.
2. Microcapsules are a way to transform gasses and liquids into solid particles.
3. It is possible to modify the surface and colloidal properties of different active agents.
4. Alter and postpone the release of medication from various pharmacological dose forms.
5. Encapsulated active agents or core materials can be modified or their release delayed to provide prolonged controlled release dosage forms.

Disadvantages of microencapsulation:
- Expensive techniques.
- Reduction in shelf-life of hygroscopic agents.
- The release of materials enclosed might be affected by the unevenness of the microencapsulation coating.

Methods of microencapsulation:

Air suspension:

The process of microencapsulation using air suspension involves scattering solids and particulate core materials in an air stream that provides support, followed by spray coating the air suspended particles (Fig.). Particulate core materials are suspended in an upward-moving air stream within the coating chamber. The coating-zone section of the coating chamber, where a coating substance is sprayed onto the moving particles, is where the chamber's design and operating characteristics affect the particle flow that is re-circulating.

Depending on the goal of microencapsulation, the core material acquires a coat during each pass through the coating-zone. This cyclic procedure is repeated. During the encapsulation process, the product is dried by the supporting air stream.

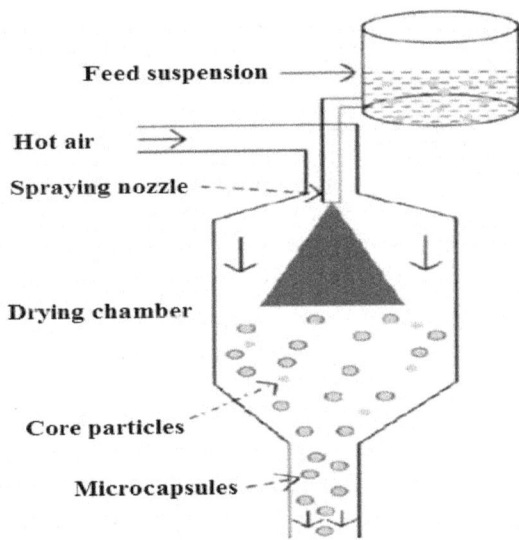

Fig: Air suspension method for microencapsulation

Coacervation phase separation:

Microencapsulation by coacervation phase separation method consists of 3 steps:

- Formationof3immisciblephases:A liquid manufacturing phase, a core material phase and a coating material phase.
- Deposition of the liquid polymer coating on the core material.
- Rigidizing the coating usually by thermal, cross linking or desolvation techniques to form microcapsules.

The liquid polymer coating that is deposited around the interface that forms between the liquid vehicle phase and the core material (Fig.). Phase separation of the polymers can frequently be brought about by inducing physical or chemical changes in the coated polymer solutions. A two phase liquid-liquid system will result from the formation and coalescence of droplets of concentrated polymer solutions. It is possible to add the coating material directly if it is an immiscible polymer. Moreover, monomers may dissolve in the liquid vehicle phase and then undergo interface polymerization. Jacketed tanks equipped with variable speed agitators are essential pieces of equipment required for microencapsulation using the coacervation phase separation method.

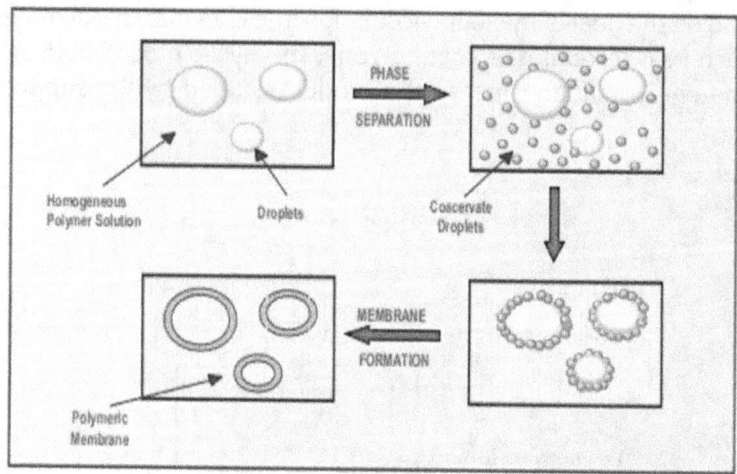

Fig.3: Coacervation phase separation method for microencapsulation

Pan coating:

The pan coating procedure, which is extensively utilized in the pharmaceutical sector to prepare controlled release particulates, can be used to microencapsulate relatively big particles, larger than 600 μ in size. This process involves coating different spherical core materials, such nonpareil sugar seeds, with a range of polymers (Fig. 4). In actual use, the coating is sprayed over the required solid core material in the coating pan in the form of an atomized spray or as a solution. In order to remove the coating solvent, heated air is typically passed over the coated materials as the coatings are applied in the coating pans. The final solvent elimination step is sometimes completed in the drying oven.

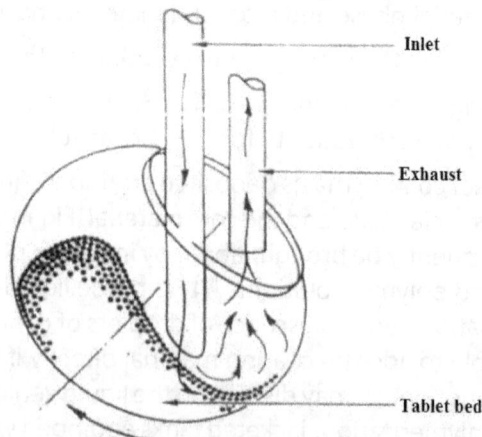

Fig.4: *Pan coating method for microencapsulation*

Micro Encapsulation

Fluidized-bed technology

Solid core materials, including liquids absorbed into porous solids, can be microencapsulated using the fluidized-bed technology approach. Medicines are encapsulated using this microencapsulation technique on a large scale. After being suspended in an air jet, solid particles that need to be enclosed are sprayed with a liquid coating substance. The capsules are transported to a location where cooling or solvent vaporization will solidify their shells. The procedures of suspending, spraying, and chilling are carried out again until the capsule-wall reaches the required thickness. When the spray nozzle is at the bottom of the fluidized bed of particles, this is referred to as the Wurster process.

Spray drying and spray congealing:

The microencapsulation techniques of spray drying and spray congealing are nearly identical in that they involve dispersing the core material in a liquefied coating agent and spraying or introducing the core coating mixture into an environment, which influences the coating's relatively quick solidification (Fig. 5). The process used to carry out the coating solidification is the primary distinction between these two microencapsulation techniques. In the spray drying procedure, the coating material's rapid evaporation in a solvent affects the coating's solidification. In the spray congealing process, a dissolved coating is solidified by adding the coating core material mixture into a non-solvent solution, or by thermally congealing molten coating material. Soil extraction or evaporation are often used techniques to remove solvent or non-solvent from coated products.

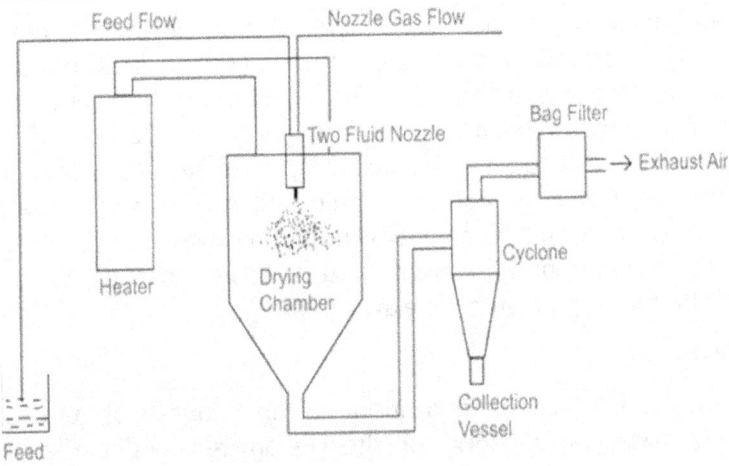

Fig.5: Spray drying method for microencapsulation

Multiorific-centrifugation

The centrifugal forces are used in the multiorific-centrifugation method of microencapsulation to propel a core particle through an enclosing membrane. The multiorific-centrifugation method involves several processing variables, such as the cylinder's rotational speed, the coating and core materials' flow rate, and the concentration, viscosity, and surface tension of the core material. Different coating materials can be used to microencapsulate liquids and solids with varying size ranges using the multiorifice-centrifugal approach. The encapsulated product may be provided as dry powder or as slurry in the hardening media.

Solvent Evaporation

The O/W emulsion, a liquid manufactured vehicle created by stirring together two immiscible liquids, is a suitable application for the solvent evaporation process. A volatile solvent that is immiscible with the liquid production vehicle phase is used to dissolve the microcapsule coating (polymer) in the solvent evaporation process. In the coating polymer solution, a core substance (drug) to be microencapsulated is dissolved or disseminated. The core-coating material mixture is agitated in the liquid manufacturing vehicle phase to produce microcapsules of the right size. System agitation is maintained until the solvent evaporates and partitions into the aqueous phase. The microcapsules produced by this method are toughened. Dispersion of the oil phase in the continuous phase can be accomplished by a variety of methods. The most popular approach involves mounting a variable speed motor to a propeller-style blade.

The rate of solvent evaporation for the coating polymer(s), temperature cycles, and agitation rates are some of the process variables that affect how dispersions are formed. The selection of the vehicle phase and solvent for the polymer coating, as well as solvent recovery systems, are the most crucial elements to take into account while preparing microcapsules using the solvent evaporation method. Many different liquid and solid core materials can be microencapsulated using the solvent evaporation process. Either water soluble or water insoluble compounds could make up the core components. As coatings, a range of film-forming polymers are available.

Polymerization:

Microencapsulation via polymerization is the process utilized to create protective microcapsule coverings on-site. The process involves the reaction of monomeric units that are positioned at the interface between a scattered core material and a continuous phase. The polymerization reaction takes place at the interfaces of liquid-liquid, liquid-gas, solid-liquid, or solid-gas because the continuous or core material supporting phase is typically a liquid or gas.

Interfacial cross-linking

A bio sourced polymer, such as a protein, takes the place of the tiny bi-functional monomer with active hydrogen atoms in the microencapsulation process known as interfacial cross-linking. The creation of a membrane results from the reaction between the acid chloride and the different functional groups of the protein at the emulsion interface. For use in pharmaceutical or cosmetic applications, the microencapsulation technique of interfacial cross-linking is incredibly flexible.

Applications:

Different applications of microencapsulation are:

1. Using microencapsulation, different sustained controlled release dosage forms can be created by altering or postponing the release of encapsulated active ingredients or core components.
2. Enteric-coated dose forms can also be created via microencapsulation, allowing the medication to be absorbed in the intestines rather than the stomach.
3. To lessen the likelihood of gastric irritation, medications that irritate the stomach are being microencapsulated.
4. The use of microencapsulation techniques can disguise the taste of bitter medication candidates.
5. Liquids and gasses can be transformed into solid particles in the form of microcapsules by the process of microencapsulation.
6. To help with the addition of oily medications to tablet dosage forms and to help with direct compression, microencapsulation can be utilized.
7. The volatility can be reduced by using microencapsulation. Volatile materials that are microencapsulated can be kept for extended periods of time without experiencing significant evaporation.
8. The encapsulated active substances are protected against a variety of environmental factors by microencapsulation, including light, heat, humidity, oxidation, etc.
9. By using microencapsulation, the hygroscopic properties of various core materials can be minimized.
10. Microencapsulation is a technique that can be used to separate incompatible chemicals. For instance, microencapsulation can be used to separate medicinal eutectics. In this instance, liquid production results from direct material contact. By microencapsulating the two

before combining, the incompatible aspirin-chlorpheniramine maleate mixture can be stabilized more effectively.

11. Microencapsulation is used to lessen the potential danger of toxic substance handling. The toxicity owing to handling of herbicides, insecticides, pesticides and fumigants, etc.

References

Allen LV, Popovich NG, Ansel HC. Pharmaceutical Dosage Forms and Drug Delivery Systems. Delhi, India: BI Publication; 2005.

Benita S. Micro encapsulation: Methods and Industrial applications, Marcel Dekker, Inc., NewYork,1996.

KiyoyamaS, ShiomoriK, KawanoY, HatateY.Preparation of micro capsules and control of their morphology. J Micro encapsulation. 2003; 20:497

Lachman LA, Liberman HA, Kanig JL. The Theory and Practice of Industrial Pharmacy.

Mumbai, India: Varghese Publishing House,1976.

Sachan NK, Singh B, Rao KR. Controlled drug delivery through micro encapsulation. Malaysian J Pharm Sci .2006; 4:65–81.

Singh MN, g Hemant KS, Ram M, Shiva kumar HG. Micro encapsulation: A promising technique for controlled drug delivery. ResPharmSci. 2010; 5(2): 65-77.

Chapter 4
Mucosal Drug Delivery system

Mucosal medication delivery systems have gained a lot of popularity in recent years. Some medications are ineffective because of reduced bioavailability, gastrointestinal intolerance, irregular and unpredictable absorption, or pre-systemic removal of alternative delivery routes. Mucosal medication administration can occur through a variety of pathways, such as buccal, ocular, nasal, and pulmonary. Typically, mucosal drug Delivery systems can be classified as:

Non-attached mucosal drug delivery systems:

These systems are designed to be absorbed through the mouth cavity's mucosa. Sublingual, quickly dissolving (melt-in-mouth, orally disintegrating) pills are a few examples.

Attached or immobilized mucosal drug delivery systems:

These systems are designed with adhesive qualities to keep them bonded to the mucosal surface. Mucoadhesive systems are another name for these systems. Examples include medicine delivery systems for the mouth, throat, vagina, nose, and throat, among others.

Various approaches have been used to achieve regulated mucosal delivery, and they are predicated on:

- Prolong duration of absorption process.
- Developing unidirectional delivery systems
- Preparing user-friendly mucosal delivery systems.

Bioadhesion

Materials that bind or cling to biological substrates are referred to as "bioadhesive" materials. A substance that interacts with biological material and is able to stick to or hold it together for a long time is referred to as "bioadhesive." Three mechanisms may lead to "bioadhesion":

a. Bioadhesion between biological layers when no artificial materials are used.
b. Adhesion of the cells to the culture dishes or to different materials, including metals, wood, and other synthetic materials.
c. The adherence of synthetic materials to biological substrates is analogous to the adherence of hydrophilic polymers to human skin or other soft tissues.

Mucoadhesive drug delivery systems

Mucoadhesive drug delivery methods make use of a polymer's mucoadhesion or bioadhesion, which becomes adhesive during hydration and allows a medicine to be targeted to a specific area of the body for a prolonged amount of time. Both systemic and local drug bioavailability greatly benefit from the capacity to keep a delivery system in place for an extended amount of time. Medicine delivery systems that are mucoadhesive make it possible to prevent the medicine from being destroyed by the contents of the stomach or from being inactivated by the liver's first pass. Mucoadhesive medication delivery systems are being developed using a variety of mucoadhesive polymers. These are often classified as:

Principles of bioadhesion / mucoadhesion: There are three steps involved in bioadhesion and mucoadhesion:

- A close bond between a membrane and a bioadhesive or mucoadhesive, either from the bioadhesive or mucoadhesive swelling or from a thorough wetting of the bioadhesive or mucoadhesive and the membrane.
- The bioadhesive or mucoadhesive enters the tissue and penetrates. Low chemical bonding can then settle after mucous interpenetrates the chains of bioadhesives and mucoadhesives.

Several theories have been proposed to explain the fundamental mechanism of bioadhesion /mucoadhesion:

a. Wetting theory: The capacity of bioadhesive and mucoadhesive polymers to diffuse and form an instantaneous bond with mucous membranes.
b. Electronic theory: Attractive electrostatic interactions between the bioadhesive/mucoadhesive polymers and the glycoprotein mucin network.

c. Adsoption theory: Chemical bonding is the outcome of surface forces, including van der Waals' forces, ionic bonds, hydrogen bonds, and covalent bonds.
d. Diffusion theory: Mucin strands physically entangled with the flexible polymeric chain.
e. Fracture theory: Examines the highest tensile stress that occurs when mucoadhesive or bioadhesive medication delivery systems separate from mucosal surfaces.

Advantages and Disadvantages

Advantages:
1. These systems permit the development of mucoadhesion, or bioadhesion, between the dosage forms and the mucosa.
2. A high drug concentration can be sustained for an extended amount of time at the absorptive surface.
3. Specific immobilization of dosage forms can occur at any location on the gingival, sublingual, buccal, or oral mucosa, among other mucosa..

Disadvantages:
1. Small mucosal surface for contact
2. Lack of flexibility of dosage forms
3. Difficult to achieve high drug release rates required for some drugs.
4. Extent and frequency and frequency of attachment may cause local irritation.

Transmucosal permeability

Oral mucosa is the term for the mucosal lining of the oral cavity. The buccal, sublingual, gingival, palatal, and labial mucosa are all parts of the oral mucosa. The transmucosal route has the potential to be an efficient way to deliver a range of medications due to its distinct environment. For medications that are typically subject to acid-hydrolysis in the gastrointestinal tract or substantial hepatic metabolism, the transmucosal route is appropriate because of its rich blood supply, increased bioavailability, lymphatic drainage, and direct access to systemic circulation. Moreover, the oral mucosa provides the benefit of mucoadhesion, which keeps drug delivery systems in touch with the absorptive mucosal surface for an extended length of time. This optimizes the drug concentration gradient across the mucosal membrane by reducing the number of differential paths. Consequently, because of its distinct physiological characteristics and great patient compliance potential, transmucosal medication administration has garnered special attention.

The medications that are to be taken via the transmucosal route must be liberated from their dosage forms, travel through the mucosal layers to the effective delivery site (such as the buccal or sublingual area), and then reach the systemic circulation. The transmucosal route's physiological characteristics, such as pH, enzyme activity, fluid volume, and oral mucosa permeability, are important in this process. Saliva secretion is another significant factor that affects how well transmucosal medication delivery works. The primary processes that allow different substances to enter cells are simple diffusion (either paracellular or transcellular), carrier-mediated diffusion, active transport, and endo- or pinocytosis. To further understand this effect, more research is necessary as there is currently limited information on how much this phenomena influences the effectiveness of oral transmucosal distribution from various drug delivery systems.

Transmucosal drug delivery is the process of delivering medication through the oral mucosal membranes. Depending on the features of the mouth cavity, transmucosal medication administration falls into three primary categories:

Sublingual delivery: Delivery of medications to the bloodstream through the sublingual mucosa, which is the membrane that covers the tongue's ventral surface and the floor of the mouth.

Buccal delivery: Medication delivery to the bloodstream through the buccal mucosa, or cheek lining.

Local delivery: For the treatment of diseases pertaining to the oral cavity, primarily dental stomatitis, fungal infections, gingivitis, periodontal disease, and ulcers.

Formulation considerations of buccal delivery systems

Buccal drug delivery is the transmucosal administration of medication across the buccal lining. A sizable contact surface is provided by the buccal mucosa's smooth, broad, and largely stationary surface (Fig. 6). The buccal mucosa's large contact surface aids in the quick and thorough absorption of drugs. In 1947, Orabase invented buccal medicine delivery by combining dental adhesive powder and gum tragacanth to deliver penicillin to the mouth mucosa. In comparison to other drug delivery methods; buccal drug delivery has shown to be especially helpful in recent years. These benefits include avoiding the gastrointestinal tract and hepatic portal system, increasing the bioavailability of drugs taken orally that would otherwise undergo hepatic first-pass metabolism, improving patient compliance because injections no longer cause pain, administering drugs to patients who are unconscious or incapable, being more convenient to administer than injections or oral medications, sustained drug delivery, ease of administering the medication, and the ability to stop the delivery of the drug by simply removing the dosage form.

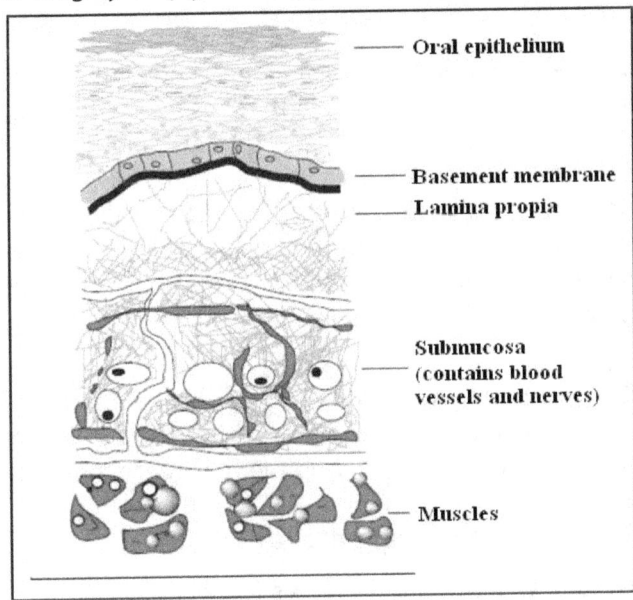

Fig.6: Schematic diagram of buccal mucosa

Buccal medication distribution takes place in a tissue that is less variable between patients and more porous than skin, which reduces inter-subject variability. Buccal drug delivery can also be utilized to transport bigger molecules, including low molecular weight heparin, due to increased mucosal permeability. Buccal drug delivery devices may also be employed to administer medications with poor or inconsistent bioavailability; additionally, pharmaceuticals with significant first-pass metabolism will have increased bioavailability. A rising number of potent peptide and protein medication molecules may be delivered via buccal administration since medicine taken from the oral cavity bypasses both first-pass metabolism and enzymatic/acid destruction in the gastrointestinal tract. Furthermore, further study on buccal delivery of these therapeutic compounds has promise for developing non-invasive alternative delivery methods.

The novel type buccal dosage forms include:
1. Buccal mucoadhesive tablets,
2. Buccal patches and films,
3. Semisolids (ointments and gels) and powders

Buccal mucoadhesive tablets: Dry dose forms known as buccal mucoadhesive tablets require moistening before being applied to the buccal mucosa.

Buccal patches and films: Buccal patches and films are made of two laminates: an impermeable backing sheet that has been cut into the necessary round or oval shape is covered with an aqueous solution of the adhesive polymer. These are also superior than creams and ointments because they deliver a precisely calibrated dosage of medication to the affected area. The most emphasis has been paid to buccal patches and films in recent years for the delivery of medications. When compared to tablets, they exhibit higher patient compliance because of their physical flexibility, which only slightly irritates the patient.

Semisolids (ointments and gels): Solid bioadhesive dosage forms are more patient-acceptable than bioadhesive gels or ointments, and the majority of the dosage forms are limited to localized drug therapy inside the mouth cavity.

Structure and Design of buccal patches

Buccal patches are of two types on the basis of their release characteristics:
1. Unidirectional buccal patches
2. Bidirectional buccal patches

Unidirectional patches release the drug only in to the mucosa, while bidirectional patches release drug in both the mucosa and the mouth.

Buccal patches are structurally of two types:

Matrix type: The medication, adhesive, and additives are combined in the matrix arrangement of the buccal patch (Fig. 7)

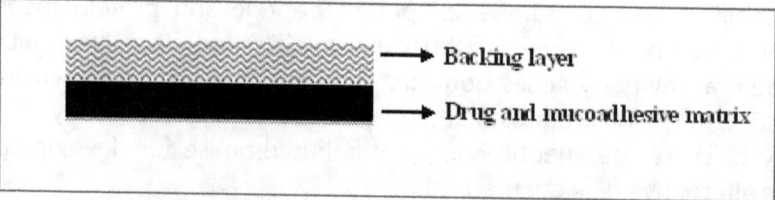

Fig 7: Schematic representation of the matrix-type buccal patch design

Reservoir type: The medicine and additives are kept apart from the adhesive in a hollow in the reservoir-designed buccal patch. To regulate the direction of drug distribution, minimize patch deformation and disintegration while in the mouth, and avoid drug loss, an impermeable backing is used.

Composition of buccal patches

Drugs: The pharmacokinetic characteristics of the medications to be supplied should be taken into consideration when choosing an appropriate medicine for the design of buccal drug delivery systems. The drug should have following characteristics for the designing of effective buccal patches:

a. The conventional single dose of the drug should be small.
b. The drugs having biological half-life between 2-8 h are good candidates for controlled drug delivery.
c. Tmax of the drug shows wider-fluctuations or higher values when given orally.
d. Through oral route drug may exhibit first pass effect or pre-systemic drug elimination.
e. The drug absorption should be passive when given orally.
f. Buccal adhesive drug delivery systems with the size 1–3 cm2 and a daily dose of 25 mg or less are preferable.

Polymers (adhesive layer): A significant component of the design of buccal patches is bioadhesive polymers. Bioadhesive polymers belong to the most varied class of polymers and offer significant advantages for patient care and treatment. By allowing the dose form to be retained at the buccal mucosal surface, these polymers provide for close contact between the absorbing tissue and the dosage form. Either polymer breakdown, diffusion, or a combination of the two can release a drug from a polymeric substance. The most common methods of polymer degradation are hydrolysis or enzymes, which can result in surface or bulk erosion. The following qualities of a perfect bioadhesive polymer for buccal patches:

a. The polymer should be inert and compatible with the buccal environment.
b. It should allow easy incorporation of drug in to the formulation.
c. The polymer and its degradation products should be non-toxic absorbable from the mucous layer.
d. It should adhere quickly to moist tissue surface and should possess the site specificity.

e. It should form a strong non-covalent bond with the mucine or epithelial surface and should possess sufficient mechanical strength.
f. The polymer must not decompose on storage or during the shelf life of the dosage form.
g. It must have high molecular weight and narrow distribution.
h. The polymer should be easily available in the market and economical.
i. The polymer should have good spread ability, wetting, swelling and solubility and biodegradability properties.
j. The pH of the polymer should be biocompatible and should possess good viscoelastic properties.
k. It should demonstrate local enzyme inhibition and penetration enhancement properties.
l. It should demonstrate acceptable shelf life.

Backing layer: The backing layer is crucial to the buccal patches' adhesion to the mucous membrane. The backing membrane's components should be inert, impermeable to the medication, and enhancer of penetration. On buccoadhesive patches, such an impenetrable film prohibits the medication loss and provides improved patient adherence. Commonly utilized components of backing membranes include ethylcellulose, Eudrajit RL and RS, and other water-insoluble polymers.

Penetration enhancer: Permeation enhancers are substances that make the buccal mucosa easier to penetrate. The physicochemical characteristics of the medication, the place of administration, the kind of vehicle, and additional excipients all influence the choice of permeation enhancer and how effective it is. When creating buccal patches, penetration enhancers need to be non-irritating and have a reversible impact. The medicine should be absorbed, and then the epithelium should regain its barrier qualities. The most prevalent groups of substances that improve buccal penetration include alcohols, bile salts, surfactants, and fatty acids, which work by interfering with the intercellular lipid packing.

Plasticizers: Appropriate plasticizers must be included to the formulation of buccal patches in order to provide the proper plasticity. Plasticizers are usually applied at a concentration of 0–20% w/w of dry polymer. Plasticizer, a crucial component of the film, lowers the glass transition temperature of the film, increasing its flexibility and lessening its bitterness. The kind of solvent used in the film casting process and the plasticizer's compatibility with the polymer determine which one to use. The mechanical properties of the film are impacted by poor use of plasticizers, thus it is important to choose them properly. Plasticizers like PEG100, 400, propylene glycol, glycerol, castor oil, etc. are frequently employed in buccal patches and films.

Taste masking agents: If the medications have a bitter taste, the formulation should include taste masking agents or techniques to conceal the harsh taste, as the bitter drugs make the formulation unappealing, especially for pediatric preparations. Therefore, the taste must be covered up before adding the medications to the buccal patches. The formulation's palatability can be increased by a number of techniques, including complexation and salting out technologies.

Mechanism of buccal absorption

Passive diffusion of the non-ionized species across the intercellular spaces of the epithelium, principally regulated by a concentration gradient, causes buccal absorption, which proceeds through the buccal mucosa and leads to systemic or local activity. The major mode of transport is the passive movement of non-ionic species over the buccal cavity's lipid membrane. Like with many other mucosal membranes, the buccal mucosa has been described as a lipoid barrier to drug passage; the more lipo-phillic the drug molecule, the more easily it is absorbed.

Factors affecting buccal absorption:

The oral cavity presents a difficult drug delivery environment due to the numerous independent and interdependent variables that lower the absorbable concentration at the absorption site.

1. **Membrane Factors:** This includes the lamina propria, intercellular lipids of the epithelium, surface area accessible for absorption, mucus layer of the salivary pellicle, and degree of keratinization. The thickness of the absorptive membrane, lymphatic and blood supply, cell renewal, and enzyme content will also help to lower the quantity and pace at which the drug enters the systemic circulation.
2. **Environmental Factors:**
a. **Saliva:** Salivary pellicle or film is the term for the thin layer of saliva that covers the buccal mucosa lining. Salivary film has a thickness of 0.07–0.10 mm. The rate of buccal absorption is influenced by the film's thickness, content, and mobility.
b. **Salivary glands:** The buccal mucosa's deep or epithelial area contains the small salivary glands. On the buccal mucosa's surface, they

continuously release mucus. Mucus may act as a barrier to medication penetration even though it aids in the retention of mucoadhesive dose forms.

Manufacturing methods of buccal patches

Manufacturing processes involved in making buccal patches, are namely solvent casting, hot melt extrusion and direct milling.

1. **Solvent casting**: Using this technique, the medication and all patch excipients are co-dispersed in an organic solvent and coated on a release liner sheet. Once the solvent has evaporated, the coated release liner sheet is bonded with a layer of protective backing material to create a laminate that can be die-cut to create patches with the correct size and shape.

2. **Hot melt extrusion**: A hot melt extrusion process involves melting a mixture of pharmaceutical materials and forcing it through an opening to produce a more uniform substance in various forms, including tablets, granules, and films. Oral disintegrating films, pellets, and granules with controlled release matrix have all been produced via hot melt extrusion. Nevertheless, the production of mucoadhesive buccal patches using hot melt extrusion has only been documented in a handful of articles.

3. **Direct milling**: In this, solvents are not used in the manufacturing process of patches. Excipients and drugs are mechanically combined by kneading or direct grinding, typically in the absence of liquids. The resulting material is rolled on a release liner until the required thickness is reached after the mixing process. Next, the backing material is laminated in the manner previously mentioned. The solvent-free procedure is chosen since there is no chance of residual solvents and no associated health risks with solvent use, even though there are very slight or nonexistent changes in patch performance between patches created by the two methods.

Advantages of buccal drug delivery systems

a. Sustained drug delivery.
b. A more convenient way to administer medications.
c. Outstanding ease of access.
d. Drug absorption by passive diffusion

e. Minimal enzyme activity, compatibility with medications or excipients that cause temporary or minor mucosal damage or irritation, ease of administration, simple drug withdrawal, and ability to penetrate.
f. Flexibility in creating release systems that can be designed in either a multidirectional or unidirectional manner for localized or systemic effects, etc.
g. The medication is shielded from deterioration by the middle gastrointestinal tract's pH and digesting enzymes.
h. Higher levels of patient adherence.
i. If therapy needs to be stopped, the formulation can be removed and a reasonably quick commencement of action can be accomplished compared to the oral route.
j. Flexibility in terms of surface, size, form, and condition.
k. Drugs from the buccal systems can be quickly absorbed into the venous system beneath the oral mucosa because the buccal mucosa is well vascularized, although being less permeable than the sublingual area.
l. Transmucosal administration is associated with less inter-patient variations, leading to reduced inter-subject variability than transdermal patches.

Limitations of buccal drug delivery systems

The following list of difficulties can be encountered while administering medication by buccal drug delivery, depending on whether systemic or local action is necessary:

a. For local effect, frequent dosage may be necessary due to the medicines' quick clearance from the body through salivary flushing or meal consumption.
b. When medications are released via a solid or semisolid delivery mechanism, their distribution inside saliva may not be uniform, which could result in some parts of the oral cavity not receiving effective quantities of the drug.
c. Patient acceptance in terms of taste, irritancy, and "mouth feel" is a problem for both local and systemic treatment.

References

Ahuja A, Khar RK, AliJ. Mucoadhesive drug delivery systems. Drug Dev Ind Pharm,1997;23 (5):489–515.

Boylan JC. Drug delivery buccal route. In: James Swarbrick, editor. Encyclopedia of Pharmaceutical Technology: Supplement 3, Marcel Dekker Inc 2001,pp.800-811.

Chien YW. Novel Drug Delivery Systems, 2nd Ed, New York: Marcel Dekker Inc.:NewYork,2007.

Gandhi RB, Robinson JR. Oral cavity as a site for bioadhesive drug delivery,Adv. DrugDel.Rev.1994;13:43-74.

Gilles P, Ghazali FA, Rathbone J. Systemic oral mucosal drug delivery systems and delivery systems, in: Rathbone M.J. (ed.), Oral Mucosal Drug Delivery, Vol. 74, Marcel DekkerInc, NewYork,1996,pp.241-285.

Hunt G, Kearney P, Kellaway IW. Mucoadhesive polymers in drug delivery systems. In: Johnson P, Lloyed-JonesJG(sds), Drug Delivery System: Fundamental and Techniqes. Elis Horwood, Chichester,1987,pp.180.

JainNK.Controlled and Novel Drug Delivery, 1st edition, published by CBS Publishers and Distributors, New Delhi. 1997.

Kamath KR, Park K. Mucosal adhesive preparations, In: Swarbrick J, Boylan JC(eds)., Encyclopedia of Pharmaceutical Technology, vol. 10., Marcel Dekker, NewYork:1994,pp.133–163.

Mathiowitz E, Chickering D, Jacob JS, Santos C. Bioadhesive drug delivery systems.In: Mathiowitz E(ed), Encyclopedia of Controlled Drug Delivery, vol.1. Wiley, NewYork,1999,pp.9–44.

Siegel IA. Permeability of the oral mucosa, In: MeyerJ. The Structure and Function of Oral Mucosa, New York: Pergamon Press,1984,pp.95-108.

Woodley J. Bioadhesion: New Possibilities for Drug Administration. Clin Pharma cokinet, 2001;40(2): 77-84.

Chapter 5
Transdermal Drug Delivery Systems

Introduction

Transdermal drug delivery systems (TDDS), sometimes referred to as "patches," are dosage forms intended to distribute a medication dosage that is therapeutically efficacious through a patient's skin. TDD is a painless way to apply a medication formulation to healthy, unbroken skin in order to administer the medicine systemically. Without building up in the dermal layer, the medication first enters the stratum corneum before moving on to the deeper layers of the epidermis and dermis. A medication can be absorbed systemically by the dermal microcirculation once it has reached the dermal layer.

Transdermal administration offers a significant advantage over oral and injectable methods due to its ability to prevent first pass metabolism and increase patient compliance, respectively. In addition to enabling continuous administration of medications with brief biological half-lives, transdermal distribution also prevents pulsed entrance into systemic circulation, which frequently results in undesired side effects.

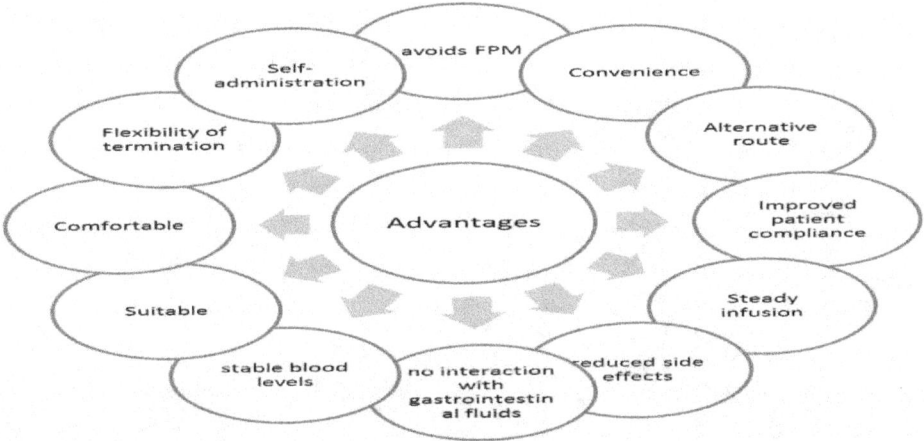

Advantages of Transdermal Drug Delivery System

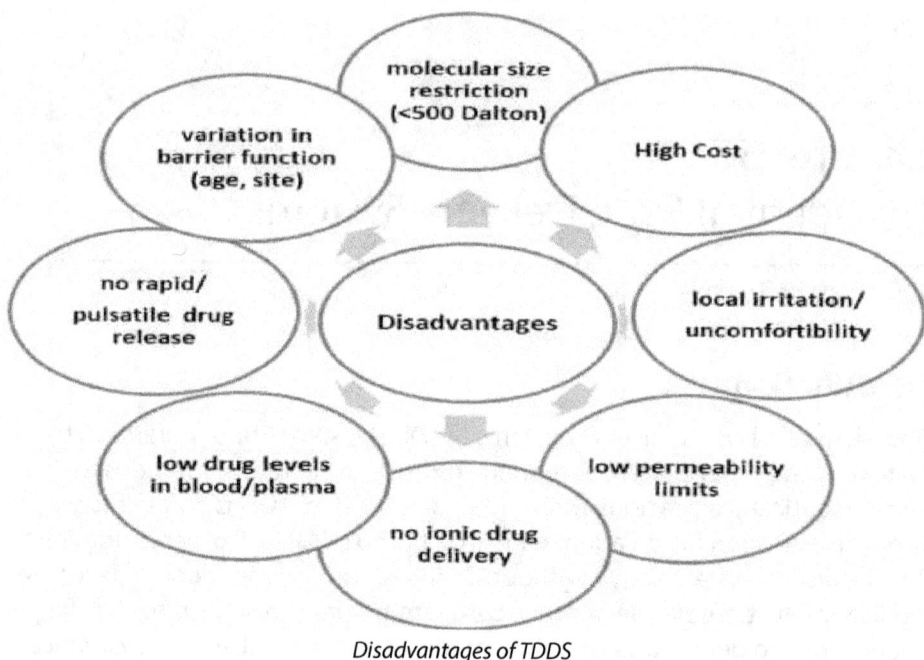

Disadvantages of TDDS

Permeation through skin

It is essential to comprehend the fundamentals of skin anatomy in order to maximize the existing potential of TDDS. The skin is a multilayered organ with numerous histological layers. The epidermis, dermis, and hypodermis are the three main divisions of the skin, arranged from top to bottom.

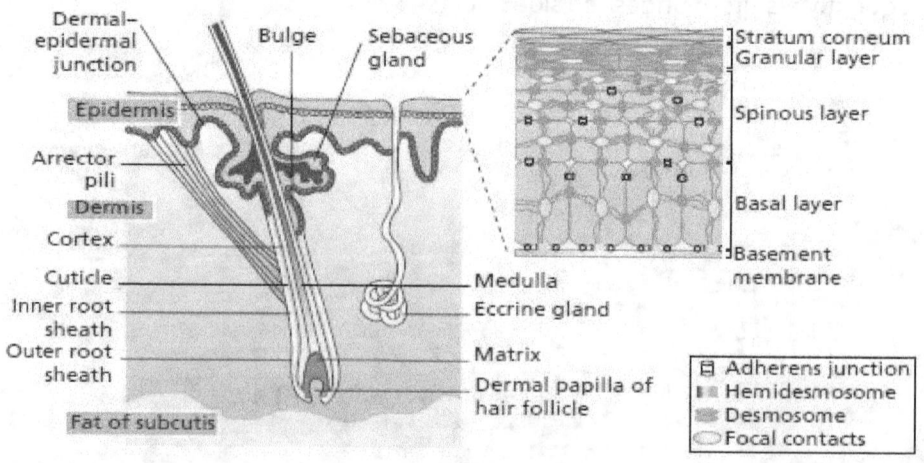

Fig: Permeation through Skin

Anatomy of Skin

Epidermis

Squamous, stratified epithelium that keratinizes. The majority of cells (>90%) are made up of keratinocytes, which are also in charge of the development of barrier function. As keratinocytes migrate to the surface of the skin, they undergo physical features such as form and size changes. The stratum corneum (SC), the outermost layer of the epidermis that is exposed to the outside world, is the fifth anatomical layer that makes up the epidermis when viewed under a microscope. These layers range in thickness from 100 to 150 micrometers. The nature of this layer makes it the most crucial for transdermal distribution since it keeps water in the body and foreign things out. Large, flat, polyhedral, plate-like envelopes that are packed with keratin and derived from dead cells that have moved up from the stratum granulosum are known as stratum granulosum (SC). The SC is made up of 10–15 layers of corneocytes, and when it's dry, its thickness is between 10–15 µm and when it's wet, 40 µm.

Dermis

Hair follicles, sweat glands, and tiny blood vessels are examples of the vast microvasculature network structures that make up the dermis. Drug delivery through the skin, therefore, requires the medication to cross the epidermis and enter the dermis, where it can be absorbed by capillaries and enter the circulatory system. The 90% of the skin's inner, bigger layer is made up mostly of connective tissue, which supports the skin's epidermal layer. Large drug molecules and cells are physically blocked by the dermal-epidermal junction, which is the line separating the dermis from the epidermis layer. It includes nerve terminals as well as lymphatic and blood vesicles. Papillary dermis and reticular dermis are the two anatomical regions that make up the dermis. The thinner outermost layer of the dermis is called the papillary. In the papillary region, collagen and elastin fibers are primarily vertically orientated and attached to the dermal-epidermal junction.

Hypodermis

The third layer below the dermis is called the subcutaneous layer, or hypodermis in histology. Huge amounts of fat cells make up the elastic subcutaneous layer, which acts as a shock absorber for blood arteries and nerve endings. This layer ranges in thickness from 4 to 9 mm on average. The exact thickness, however, varies from person to person and is dependent upon the specific body area.

A molecule comes into contact with sebum, natural microbial flora, cellular detritus, and other things when it reaches undamaged skin.

Routes of skin penetration

Transcellular transport is the primary mode of transport for compounds soluble in water. It involves the stratum corneum's lipid structure and passage into the cytoplasm of corneocytes9. Lipid soluble compounds are transported through an intercellular channel that appears to involve the endogenous lipid in the stratum corneum. The trans-epidermal route, as illustrated below, refers to the combination of the transcellular and intercellular pathways.

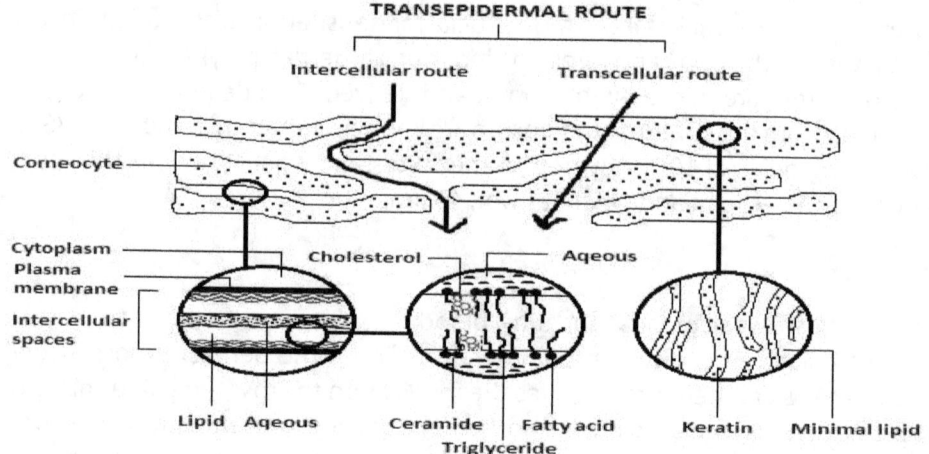

Fig: Transdermal Route

Solute molecules can enter the skin by the sweat duct, sebaceous glands, or hair follicles. The terms "shunt" and "appendageal route" refer to these passageways collectively. It is widely acknowledged that the fractional area for medication absorption in the skin appendages is roughly 0.1%. Therefore, rather than concentrating on the appendages, the key goal is to create penetration strategies through the stratum corneum.

The dead cells of the SC are the primary obstacles to absorption because they limit the passage of pharmacological molecules both inward and outward and have a high electrical resistance. The SC is made up of flattened keratinized cells and is a heterogeneous tissue. Compared to the cells next to the underlying granular layer, these cells' outer layers are less densely packed. The epidermal barrier thus becomes increasingly impermeable in the lower part, and this feature has given rise to the theory that there is a distinct barrier—the so-called SC—at this level. Therefore, the SC serves as the rate-limiting barrier, or the tissue

that offers the greatest resistance to the passage of molecules, as they enter the skin from the environment. **Transdermal permeation or percutaneous absorption can be seen as a combination of several processes after the dose form is administered topically.**
  a. Adsorption of a penetrated molecule on to the surface layers of SC.
  b. Diffusion through SC and through viable epidermis.

Percutaneous Absorption

It is a step-wise process of penetration of substances in to various layers of skin and permeation across the skin in to systemic circulations and can be divided in to three parts:
  a. **Penetration:** the entry of a substance in to a particular layer.
  b. **Permeation:** the penetration from one layer in to another, and is different both functionally and structurally from the first layer.
  c. **Absorption:** the uptake of a substance in to systemic circulation.

Factors affecting Permeation

Passive diffusion, mainly via the trans-epidermal route in a steady state or the trans-appendageal route in an initially non-steady state, is the primary mode of transport across mammalian skin. The following three categories comprise the variables that influence the skin's permeability**:**

Physicochemical properties of the permeate molecule

Partition co-efficient: Drugs that are soluble in both lipids and water are more readily absorbed via the skin. The partition co-efficient exhibits a linear effect on the transdermal permeability co-efficient. A medicinal molecule's lipid/water partition coefficient may change if the vehicle is changed. Chemical alteration of a drug molecule can change its partition co-efficient without impacting the medication's pharmacological action.
  1. Molecular size: The transdermal flow and the molecule's molecular weight have an inverse relationship. The medication molecules that are chosen as potential transdermal delivery options often fall into a small molecular weight range (100-500 Dalton).
  2. Solubility / Melting point: Transdermal candidates should have lipophilicity because lipophilic molecules tend to penetrate the skin more quickly than hydrophilic ones. Medications with high melting points are not very soluble in water at room temperature and pressure.

3. PH condition: Medications that are acidic or basic are more quickly absorbed when their pH is lower, while medications that remain stable have a higher penetration rate. Movement of ionizable organisms demonstrates a significant pH dependence from aqueous solutions. The pH partition hypothesis states that only the unionized version of the medication has a substantial chance of passing through the lipid barrier.

A. Physicochemical properties of the drug delivery system:

i. The affinity of the vehicle for the drug molecules:

It may have an impact on how the medication molecule is released from the carrier. The drug's release rate is determined by its solubility in the carrier. The medication's dissolution or suspension in the delivery/carrier system and its interfacial partition coefficient from the delivery system to epidermal tissue determine the drug release mechanism.

ii. Composition of drug delivery system:

The drug delivery system's composition may have an impact on the SC's permeability through hydration in addition to the drug release rate.

iii. Enhancement of transdermal permeation:

The medicine releases less from the dosage form as a result of the dead nature of the SC. Hence, penetration enhancers have the ability to alter the physicochemical or physiological makeup of SC and boost the drug's skin penetration. It is discovered that a variety of chemical compounds have this medication penetration-enhancing ability.

B. Physiological and pathological condition of the skin:

a. Skin age:

Water permeation has been demonstrated to be the same in adults and children, but fetal and newborn skin appears to be more permeable than mature adult skin. As a result, topical steroid absorption occurs more quickly in children than in adults through the skin.

b. Lipid film:

The excretion of sebaceous glands leaves a thin lipid film on the skin's surface, and cell lipids like sebum and epidermal cells—which contain emulsifying agents—may create a protective layer to stop the skin's natural moisturizing factor from being removed and support the preservation of the SC's barrier function.

c. Skin hydration:
Hydrating SC can improve permeability through the skin. The investigation on the rate of penetration of salicylic acid through skin with hydrated and dry corneum revealed that the most water-soluble esters penetrated the tissues more quickly when the tissues were hydrated than when the other esters did.

d. Skin temperature:
The rate of skin penetration increases with increased skin temperature. An increase in skin temperature may also cause blood vessels that are in contact with the skin to dilate more widely, increasing the rate of absorption through the skin.

e. Cutaneous drug metabolism:
Because metabolic enzymes are present in the layers of skin, some of the medicine that has crossed the SC barrier and entered the general circulation is inactive or metabolic. Over 95% of the absorbed testosterone was said to be digested as it was expressed through the skin.

f. Species differences:
The thickness of the stratum corneum, the quantity of sweat glands, and the quantity of hair follicles per unit surface area are only a few examples of the anatomical variances seen in the skin of mammals from various species.

g. Pathological injury to the skin:
Skin injuries can disrupt the continuity of the SC and increase the permeability of the skin.

Permeation Enhancers

These substances change the skin's ability to act as a barrier to the flow of a desired penetrant, therefore promoting skin permeability. Penetration enhancers are added to a formulation to increase the drug's diffusivity and solubility through the skin, which would reversibly lower the skin's barrier resistance. Consequently, the medication is able to permeate living tissues and enter the bloodstream.

The flux J of drug across the skin can be written as

$J = D \, [dc/dx]$

J=The Flux,

D=diffusion coefficient,

C=Concentration of the diffusing species,

X =Spatial coordinate.

The methods employed for modifying the barrier properties of the SC to enhance the drug penetration (and absorption) through the skin can be categorized as chemical and physical methods of enhancement.

Chemical Enhancers

Chemical permeation enhancers can work by one or more of the following three principle mechanisms:

- Relaxation of the extremely ordered lipid structure of the stratum corneum.
- Interacting with aqueous domain of bilayer of lipid.
- Enhanced partition of the drug, by addition of co enhancer or solvent in to the stratum corneum.
- Promoting penetration and establishing drugs reservoir in the stratum corneum.

Chemical permeation enhancer's work by altering the skin's structure in the ways mentioned above. Different chemical permeation enhancers engage in ionic and hydrogen bonding interactions with the polar head groups. The relaxation at the head part is brought on by the subsequent rupture of the lipid hydration spheres and alteration in the characteristics of the head group. The resistances of this lipid-enriched area to polar molecules may be lessened by this relaxation. An additional factor may be a rise in the water layer's volume, which causes the tissue to receive greater water flow. Referred to as solvent swelling, which increases the cross sectional area available for polar molecule diffusion. At the lipid interface, in addition to the water in structure, some free water becomes available. Basic dehydration can potentially trigger this process. Diethyltoluamide (DEET), propylene glycol (PG), dimethyl sulfoxide (DMSO), and dimethylacetamide (DMA) are a few of the permeation enhancers that have been the subject of much research. The keratin filaments found in corneocytes can interact with penetration enhancers like DMSO, urea, and surfactants to cause internal cell disruption, which raises the diffusion coefficient and permeability.

Physical Enhancers

Electroporation

Electro-permeabilization has been used for up to a century to improve dispersion through biological barriers. Applying high-voltage pulses to the skin causes disturbance through electroporation. Most often, high voltages (≥ 100 V) and brief treatment times (milliseconds) are used. Enhancing the skin permeability of molecules with varying lipophilicity and size (small molecules, proteins, peptides, and oligonucleotides) has been accomplished with success using this method.

Iontophoresis

By applying a low-level electric current to the skin, either directly or indirectly through the dose form, this approach improves the penetration of a topically administered medicinal substance. Electro-repulsion (for charged solutes), electro-osmosis (for uncharged solutes), and electro-perturbation (for both charged and uncharged) processes may be responsible for an increase in drug permeation as a consequence of this technology, alone or in combination.

Ultrasound

Sonophoresis is a common term for ultrasound, which is the application of ultrasonic radiation to improve transdermal transport of solutes either concurrently or through pretreatment. According to one theory, the creation of gaseous holes inside intercellular lipids upon ultrasonic exposure causes disruption of the stratum corneum, which in turn accounts for the rise in skin permeability.

Magnetophoresis

Through the use of an external magnetic field as a driving factor, this technique amplifies the diffusion of a diamagnetic solute through the skin. Magnetic field exposure on the skin may potentially cause structural changes that lead to increased permeability.

Thermophoresis

People typically have a skin surface temperature of 32°C due to a variety of homeostatic mechanisms.

Micro needle-based devices

This technique provides the basis for one of the earliest patents ever submitted for a drug delivery system for the percutaneous administration of medication. These 50–110 mm long microneedles will pierce the epidermis and stratum corneum in order to transfer the medication from the reservoir.

Needle less injection

According to reports, there is no discomfort involved in applying medication topically by needleless injection. As a result, this approach does not involve the risks, discomfort, or anxiety that comes with using hypodermic needles.

Ideal properties of penetration enhancer

The ideal properties of penetration enhancers are:

- It should be pharmacologically inert.
- It is should be nontoxic, nonirritating, and non-allergenic to the skin.
- It should produce rapid onset of action; predictable and suitable duration of action for the drug used.
- Following removal of the enhancer, the stratum corneum should immediately and fully recover its normal barrier property.
- The barrier function of the skin should decrease in one direction only i.e., they should permit therapeutic agents into the body and efflux of endogenous materials should not occur.
- It should be chemically and physically compatible with the delivery system.
- It should be non-damaging to viable cells.
- They should be Inexpensive and cosmetically acceptable.
- The Penetration enhancer used should be economical.

Basic Components of TDDS

Transdermal drug delivery system consists of the following components.

1. **Polymer Matrix**: The Polymer controls their lease of the drug from the device. Possible useful polymers for transdermal devices are:
    a. **Natural Polymers:** e.g. : cellulose derivatives, Zein, Gelatin, Shellac, Waxes, Proteins, Gums and their derivatives, Natural rubber, Starch etc.

- b. **Synthetic Elastomers:** e.g.: polybutadieine, Hydrinrubber, Polysiloxane, Silicone rubber, Nitrile, Acrylonitrile, Butylrubber, Styrenebutadieine rubber, Neoprene etc.
- c. **Synthetic Polymers: e.g:** Polyvinyl chloride, Polyethylene, Polypropylene, Polyacrylate, Polyamide, Polyurea, Polyvinyl pyrrolidone, Polymethyl methacrylate, Epoxy etc.

2. **Drug**

The medicine must be carefully chosen in order to build a transdermal drug delivery system that works. Some of the desired characteristics of a medication for transdermal distribution are listed below.

Physicochemical properties:

- The B drug should have a molecular weight less than approximately 1000 Daltons.
- The drug should have affinity for both lipophilic and hydrophilic phases. Extreme partitioning characteristics are not conducive to successful drug delivery via the skin.
- The drug should have low melting point.
- Along with the properties the drug should be potent, having short half life and non-irritating.

3. **Permeation Enhancers**

These substances change the skin's ability to act as a barrier to the flow of a desired penetrant, increasing skin permeability. In order to increase a drug's diffusivity and solubility through the skin and hence reversibly lower the skin's barrier resistance, penetration enhancers are added to a formulation. Water, pyrolidones, fatty acids, alcohols, zone and its derivatives, alcohol and glycols, essential oils, terpenes and their derivatives, urea, and surfactants are among them.

4. **Pressure sensitive adhesives(PSA)**

Any transdermal device that needs to be fastened to the skin can do so by placing a PSA inside the device or on its face, then extending it outside.

- The first approach involves the development of new polymers, which include hydrogel hydrophilic polymers, and polyurethanes.
- The second strategy involves altering the chemistries of the PSAs that are currently in use, like acrylates and silicones, either chemically or physically. Physical modification is the process of

creating base adhesives with special additives that work in concert with the medicine and excipients in the system formulation to improve skin adhesion and promote drug distribution. To increase drug delivery rates, chemical modification entails grafting or chemically adding functional monomers to the traditional PSA polymers.

5. **Backings Laminates**

Laminates for backings are chosen based on their look, pliability, and occlusion requirements. Aluminum vapor coated layers, polyester, polyethylene, and polyolefin films are a few types of backings. Additional assiduities include the backing's additives seeping out and the medicine or compositions diffusing through it. An overemphasis on chemical resistance frequently results in stiffness and high air and moisture exclusivity. When used repeatedly, it raises the TDDS and could irritate the skin.

6. **Release Liner**

A protective liner that covers the patch while it is being stored is taken off and thrown away before the patch is applied to the skin. The liner should not react chemically with the TDDS because it will be in close contact with it. A base layer, such as paper fabric, may be non-occlusive or occlusive, such as polyethylene or polyvinyl chloride, and a release coating layer, consisting of silicon or Teflon, make up the release liner. Polyester foil and metalized lamination, which shields the patch from storage damage, are additional materials used to make TDDS liners. Before using, the liner is taken out.

7. **Other Excipients**

Drug reservoirs are prepared using a variety of solvents, including dichloromethane, acetone, methanol, and chloroform. To provide the transdermal patch additional plasticity, plasticizers including propylene glycol, dibutyl phthalate, trietyl citrate, and polyethylene glycol are used.

Formulation Approaches of TDDS

The different formulation approaches for TDDS are discussed as follows.

1. Polymer membrane permeation controlled TDD system:

The drug reservoir is positioned between a rate-controlling polymeric membrane and a drug-impermeable backing laminate. The drug is uniformly distributed in the drug reservoir compartment within a solid polymeric matrix (such as polyisobutylene) and suspended in an unleachable viscous liquid medium (such as silicon fluid), creating a paste-like suspension. A microporous or nonporous polymeric membrane, such as an ethylene-vinyl acetate copolymer, is used as a rate-controlling membrane. Estraderm (used twice a week to treat postmenopausal syndrome) and Duragesic (used to manage chronic pain for 72 hours) are two examples of this kind of patch.

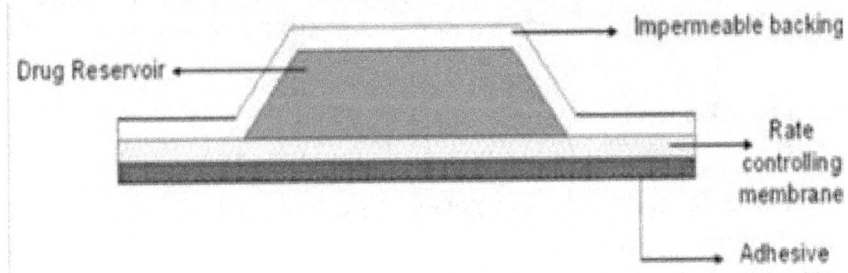

Membrane permeation controlled system.

The intrinsic rate of drug release from this type of drug delivery system is defined by:

{dq/dt}= Cr/1/Pm+1/Pa.

Where, Cr=Concentration of drug in the drug reservoir.

Pa=Permeation Co-efficient of adhesive layer.

Pm= Permeation Co-efficient of rate controlling membrane.

For any micro porous rate – controlling membrane, Pm approximately represents the sum of permeability co-efficient across the pores and polymeric material. **Pa** and **Pm** may be separately defined as **Pa**

Pa=Ka/m. Da/ha

Pm=Km/r.Dm/hm

Where,

Da=Diffusion Co-efficient

Dm=Diffusion Co-efficient of rate–controlling membrane

Ka/m=Partition Co-efficient for interfacial partitioning of drug from rate controlling membrane to adhesive layer

Km/r=Partition Co-efficient for interfacial partitioning of drug from reservoir to rate controlling membrane

hm= Thickness of rate=Controlling membrane.

Ha=Thickness of adhesive layer

2. Polymer matrix diffusion controlled TDD system:

By evenly spreading drug particles inside a hydrophilic (or lipophilic) polymer matrix, the drug reservoir is created in this way. After that, the polymer matrix is molded into discs with a predetermined surface area and thickness. After that, the medicated disc is molded into an occlusive base plate within a drug-impermeable backing compartment. Lastly, the sticky polymer is applied all the way around the film. For example, a transdermal therapeutic device that releases nitroglycerine at a daily dosage of 0.5g/cm2 is used to treat angina pectoris.

Rate of drug release in this system is given by the equation:

$q/dt = \{AC_pD_p/2t\}^{1/2}$

Where,

A=Initial drug loading dose dispersed in polymer matrix

Cp=Solubility of drug in Polymer

Dp=Diffusivity of drug in Polymer since

Cp is equal to **Cr**.

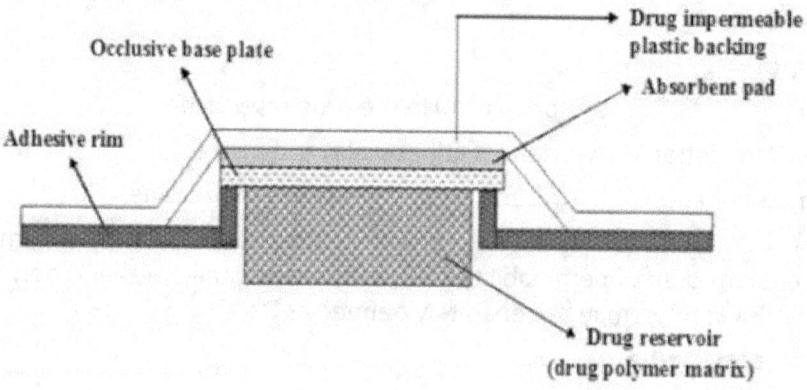

Fig: Matrix diffusion controlled Systems

3. Adhesive Dispersion–Type Systems:

This type of membrane permeation-controlled system is simplified. The medication and other carefully chosen excipients are mixed right into the glue solution in this technique. After mixing and casting them into thin films, the solvent is eventually removed by drying the film. Next, the rate-controlling adhesive polymer membrane and banking laminate are placed between the drug reservoir (film).

The rate of drug release from this system is given by,

dq/dt=Cr.Ka/r.Da/ha

Where **Ka/r** = Partition co-efficient for interfacial partitioning of drug from reservoir layer to adhesive layer.

Examples: Isosorbide dinitrate – releasing TDDS – 24 hr, Used in Angina Pectoris Verapamil –releasingTDDS–24 hrs, used in Hypertension.

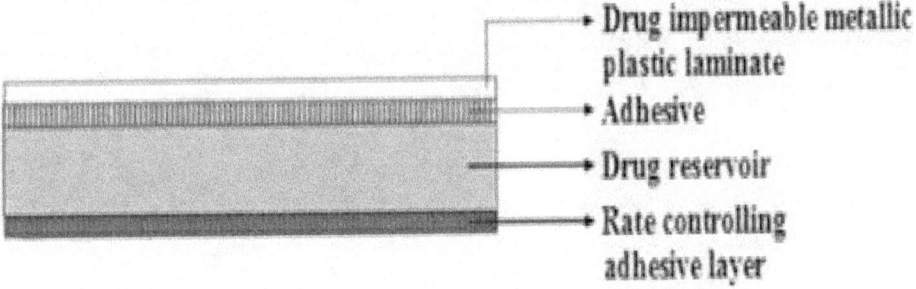

Fig: Adhesive Dispersion–Type Systems

4. Micro reservoir dissolution controlled TDD system:

It is regarded as a hybrid drug delivery device that combines matrix dispersion and reservoir technologies. This method creates thousands of unleachable microscopic drug reservoirs by first suspending the drug solids in an aqueous solution of a water-miscible drug solubilizer, such as polyethylene glycol, and then uniformly dispersing the drug suspension with a controlled aqueous soluble lipophillic polymer using high shear mechanical force.

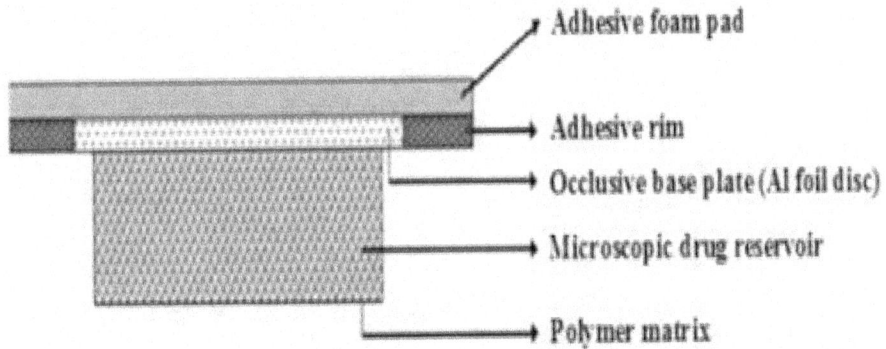

Fig: Micro-reservoir type Systems

Chapter 6
Gastro-retentive Drug Delivery System

Introduction

By extending the stomach residence period, gastro retentive drug delivery aims to target site-specific medication release in the upper gastrointestinal tract (GIT) for either local or systemic effects. The gastric retention time (GRT) of medications can be greatly extended by using gastro-retentive dose forms, which can stay in the stomach area for extended periods of time.

Drug delivery systems that are gastro-retentive offer an effective way to increase the bioavailability and regulated release of several medications. The idea of GRDDS is to extend the duration of gastric retention. Medications that need to have their bioavailability increased and their administration managed can be made using the new idea of GRDDS.

This technology is becoming more and more popular since it is affordable and simple to construct. These systems enable the use of a wide variety of medications with enhanced bioavailability. Additionally, the technology may be utilized to focus medications to specific bodily parts, such as the duodenum and stomach, for the treatment of inflammation and cancer. For patients who prefer an oral route with less frequent doses, GRDDS is an invaluable tool.

Need for gastro-retention

Drugs that are absorbed from the proximal part of the gastro intestinal tract (GIT).

- Drugs that are less soluble or that degrade at the alkaline pH.
- Drugs that are absorbed due to variable gastric emptying time.
- Local or sustained drug delivery to the stomach and proximal small intestine to treat certain conditions.
- Treatment of peptic ulcers caused by H.Pylori infections. Potential Drug Candidates for Gastro-retentive Drug Delivery Systems:

- Drugs those are locally active in the stomach.
- Drugs that have narrow absorption window in gastrointestinal tract (GIT).
- Drugs those are unstable in the intestinal or colonic environment.
- Drugs that disturb normal colonic microbes Drugs that exhibit low solubility at high pH values.

Advantages of GRDDS

- This system offers improved bioavailability
- It reduces dose and dosing frequency.
- This system minimizes fluctuation of drug concentration in blood
- This system helps in targeting of drugs
- Local action can be achieved in GIT. Eg. Antacids
- This system reduces the side effect.
- Sustained release can be achieved.
- Safest route of administration
- It is economic and can be used for wide range of drugs.

Disadvantages of GRDDS

- This system should be administered with plenty of water.
- Drugs with solubility or stability problem in GIT can't be administered.
- Drugs, which undergoes first pass metabolism, are not suitable .e.g. Nifedipine.
- Drugs which are irritant to gastric mucosa are not suitable .E.g. Aspirin & NSAID.
- Drugs that absorb equally well through GIT. E.g. Isosorbidedi nitrate, Nifidipine

Approaches for GRDDS

Different approaches of gastro-retentive drug delivery systems are discussed as follows:

1. Floating system or Low density system:

The drug is released from the system slowly and at a desired rate, increasing the gastric residence time and improving control over fluctuations in the plasma drug concentrations. After the drug is completely released, the residual system is emptied from the stomach. Floating Drug Delivery Systems (FDDS) have a bulk density lower than gastric fluids, allowing them to remain buoyant in the stomach for an extended period of time without affecting the gastric emptying rate.

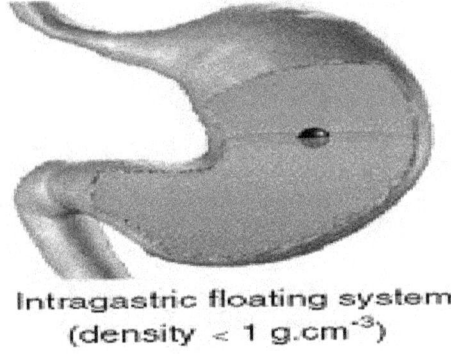

Fig: Intra Gastric Floating System

Low-density systems (Floating system)

Because floating drug delivery systems (FDDS) have a lower bulk density than gastric fluids, they float in the stomach for extended periods of time without slowing down the rate at which the stomach empties. The medicine is gradually removed from the system at the proper pace while it is floating on the contents of the stomach. The stomach is cleared of any leftover medication once the substance has been released. As a result, the variations in plasma drug concentration are better controlled and the GRT is raised. To maintain the dose form consistently buoyant on the meal's surface, however, a minimum amount of floating force (F) is also necessary, in addition to the minimal stomach content necessary to permit the correct realization of the buoyancy retention principle. A new device measures the dynamics of the floating force by calculating the resultant weight (RW). The way the RW apparatus works is that it continually measures the force (F) as a function of time needed to keep the submerged item in place.

The object floats better if RW is on the higher positive side.

RW or F= Fbuoyancy- Fgravity=(Df-Ds)gV,

Where,

RW =total vertical force,

Df=fluid density,

Ds=object density,

V=volume

g=acceleration due to gravity. Gf=gastric fluid

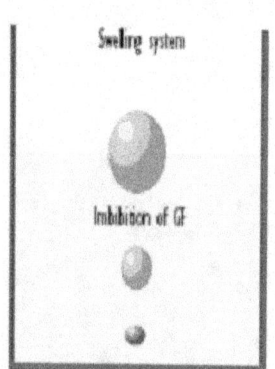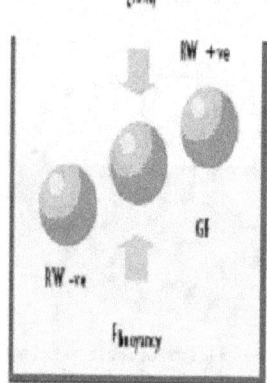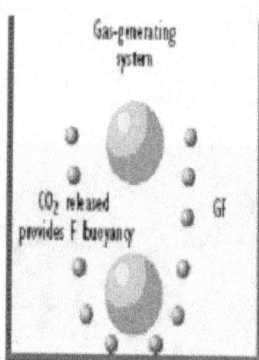

Fig: Mechanism of Floating Systems

When a system produces gas, carbon dioxide is produced, which makes the beads float in the stomach. Additionally, in non-effervescent settings, these dosage forms are buoyant due to the air retained by the inflated polymer.

Based on the mechanism of buoyancy, two different technologies have been used in development of floating drug delivery systems. These include:

a. Non-Effervescent system.
b. Effervescent system.

Non-Effervescent System

The non-effervescent FDDS is based on the polymer's swelling mechanism or bioadhesion to the GI tract's mucosal layer. The most often utilized non-effervescent excipients. FDDS include hydrophilic gums, polysaccharides, gel-forming or highly swellable cellulose hydrocolloids, and matrix-forming materials including polycarbonate, polyacrylate, polymethacrylate, and polystyrene as well as bioadhesive polymers like chitosan and carbopol.

This system can be further divided in to these-types:

a. Hydro-dynamically balanced systems.

These methods include medications with gel-forming hydrocolloids designed to float on stomach contents. These are dosage forms that come in single units and comprise one or more hydrophilic polymers that gel. Common excipients employed in the development of these systems include hydroxypropyl methylcellulose (HPMC), hydroxethyl cellulose (HEC), hydroxypropyl cellulose (HPC), sodium carboxymethyl cellulose (NaCMC), polycarbophil, polyacrylate, polystyrene, agar, carrageenans, or alginic acid. Drugs are combined with the polymer and typically given in hydrodynamically balanced system capsules. When the capsule shell comes into touch with water, it dissolves and the mixture expands to form a gelatinous barrier that gives the dose form long-lasting buoyancy in gastric juice. Because water may enter the inner layers due to constant surface erosion, surface hydration and buoyancy are maintained. Fatty excipients are used to create low-density formulations that lessen erosion. In the 1980s, the system-based Madopar LPR was sold. The balance of drug loading and the impact of the polymer on the release profile are key factors in effective drug delivery. Several approaches have been tested and studied to increase the effectiveness of the floating hydrodynamically balanced systems.

b. Microballoons /Hollow microspheres:

To extend the dosage form's gastrointestinal retention time (GRT), microballoons and hollow microspheres containing medications in their other polymer shelves were made using straightforward solvent evaporation or solvent diffusion evaporation techniques. Polycarbonate, cellulose acetate, calcium alginate, Eudragit S, agar, low methoxylated pectin, and other polymers are frequently utilized to create these systems. Polymer amount, plasticizer polymer ratio, and formulation solvent all affect buoyancy and medication release from dosage forms. For more than 12 hours, the micro-balloons remained suspended above the surface of an acidic dissolving medium that contained surfactant. Because hollow microspheres combine the benefits of superior floating and multiple-unit systems, they are now regarded as one of the most promising buoyant systems.

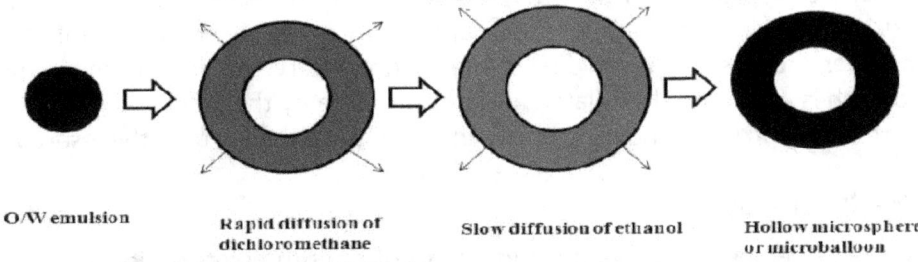

Fig: Microballoons flow for Hollow Microsphere

Effervescent System

A floating chamber, which may be filled with air, vacuum, or inert gas, can be included into a medicine delivery system to make it float in the stomach. Either an organic solvent can volatilize or an effervescent interaction between organic acids and bicarbonate salts can bring gas into a floating chamber. These effervescent systems further classified in to two types:
1. Volatile liquid or vacuum containing systems.
2. Gas generating systems.

Volatile liquid or vacuum containing systems

a. Intra gastric floating gastrointestinal drug delivery system

This system floats in the stomach because of floatation chamber, which is vacuum or filled with a harmless gas or air, while the drug reservoir is encapsulated by a micro porous compartment

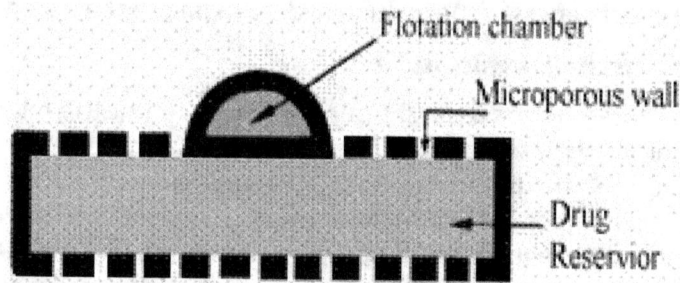

Fig: Intra-gastric floating gastrointestinal drug delivery device

b. Inflatable gastrointestinal delivery systems

An inflatable chamber that contains liquid ether and gasifies at body temperature to expand the chamber in the stomach is a feature of these devices. These systems are constructed by filling the inflated chamber with a gelatin capsule-encased drug reservoir, which may be a drug or an impregnated polymeric matrix. Following oral delivery, the capsule dissolves, releasing the inflated chamber and the drug reservoir. The medication reservoir compartment in the stomach is automatically inflated and held in place by the inflatable chamber. The medication is continually pumped into the stomach fluid from the reservoir.

Bioadhesive Systems

By strengthening the closeness and length of the drug's interaction with the biological membrane, bio/mucoadhesive systems have the ability to attach to the surface of the gastric epithelial cells or mucin, which may be used to prolong the gastro retention of drug delivery systems (DDS) in the stomach. A natural or synthetic polymer that may form an adhesive connection based on hydration-mediated, bonding-mediated, or receptor-mediated adhesion with a biological membrane or the mucous lining the gastrointestinal tract is known as a bio/muco-adhesive material.

The binding of polymers to the mucin-epithelial surface can be sub-divided in to three broad categories-

1. Hydration-mediated adhesion
2. Bonding-mediated adhesion
3. Receptor-mediated adhesion

1. **Hydration-mediated adhesion:** Certain hydrophilic polymers tend to imbibe large amount of water and become sticky, there by acquiring bioadhesive properties.
2. **Bonding-mediated adhesion:** Polymer adhesion to mucous or epithelial cell surfaces occurs through a variety of bonding methods, including as chemical and physical-mechanical bonding. The adhesive substance can form physical-mechanical linkages when it is inserted into the mucosa's folds and crevices. Chemical bonds can have two different types: main covalent bonds and secondary ionic links. Stronger specific interactions like hydrogen bonds and dispersive interactions like van der Waals interactions make up secondary chemical bonds. The hydroxyl and carboxylic groups are the hydrophilic functional groups that create hydrogen bonding.
3. **Receptor-mediated adhesion:** Dosage forms' ability to remain in the stomach is improved by certain polymers that can attach to particular receptor locations on cell surfaces. Specific interactions occur between some plant lectins, including tomato lectins, and the sugar groups found in mucus.

High Density Systems

These systems, which have a density of around 3 g/cm3, are kept in the stomach's antrum and can endure its peristaltic motions. The main significant disadvantage of these systems is their technical difficulty in producing formulations with a high drug content (>50%) and a density of around 2.5 g/cm3. Using this method, dosage forms must be formulated with a density greater than the average stomach contents (~ 1.004 gm/cm3). These formulations are made by mixing inert substances like iron powder, barium sulfate, zinc oxide, titanium oxide, etc. with the medicine or coating it on a heavy core. Density may be increased by the materials by 1.5–2.4 gm/cm³. It appears that a density of around 2.5 gm/cm3 is required to significantly extend the gastric residence duration. However, no system has been sold and the usefulness of this system in humans has not been noted.

Raft forming Systems

The administration of antacids and medications for gastrointestinal infections and illnesses has drawn a lot of interest to raft-forming mechanisms. When viscous cohesive gel comes into touch with stomach fluids, a continuous layer known as a raft is formed when each piece of the liquid expands. This is one of the mechanisms underlying the development of rafts. Because CO_2 production results in a low bulk density, this raft floats on stomach juices. To make the system less thick and allow it to float on the stomach contents, the system typically consists of an alkaline bicarbonate or carbonate responsible for the generation of CO_2 and a gel-forming agent. When in contact with stomach contents, the system's gel-forming ingredient (such as alginic acid), sodium bicarbonate, and acid neutralizer create a foamy sodium alginate gel, or raft. As a barrier between the stomach and the esophagus, the raft that has so created floats on the gastric fluids and stops the reflux of the gastric contents, or gastric acid, into the esophagus.

Application of GRDDS

Gastro-retentive drug delivery system offer several applications as follows:

1. **Bioavailability:** When compared to the administration of non-GRDDS controlled release polymeric formulations, the bioavailability of controlled release GRDDS is markedly improved. The amount of medication absorption is influenced by a number of concurrent processes that are connected to drug absorption and transit in the gastrointestinal tract.

2. **Site Specific Drug Delivery Systems:** These systems are especially useful for medications like furosemide that are selectively absorbed from the gut. The medication is delivered to the stomach gradually and under control, limiting systemic exposure while supplying adequate local therapeutic amounts. It lessens the negative impact that medications have on blood circulation. A site-directed administration system's extended stomach availability may help lessen the need for frequent dosage.

3. **Sustained Drug Delivery:** Large doses and going via the pyloric

aperture are not allowed in this system. Nicardipine hydrochloride sustained release floating capsules were created and tested in vivo. The sustained release floating capsules' plasma concentration time curves indicate a longer administration period (16 hours) than that of traditional capsules (8 hours). Because the hydrodynamically balanced system (HBS) can stay in the stomach for extended lengths of time, it may release the medication continuously for longer durations of time.

4. **Enhancement of Absorption:** In order to maximize absorption, drugs with limited bioavailability due to site-specific absorption from the upper regions of the GIT may be designed as floating drug delivery devices. These dosage forms' floating property allows them to stay in the stomach area for an extended amount of time, allowing the medication to be absorbed at its fastest pace possible.

5. **Minimize adverse activity at the colon:** The quantity of medication that enters the colon is reduced when it is retained in the HBS systems of the stomach. As a result, undesirable medication effects in the colon may be avoided. The GRDF formulation of beta lactam antibiotics, which are absorbed solely from the small intestine and whose presence in the colon causes the development of microorganism resistance, is justified by this pharmacodynamic feature.

Chapter 7
Naso-Pulmonary Drug Delivery System

Introduction

Nasal routes of drug delivery

Since the nasal mucus has a neutral pH, is less diluted by the gastrointestinal contents, and is permeable to more compounds than the gastrointestinal tract due to a lack of pancreatic and gastric enzymatic activity, the nasal route of drug delivery has been explored as a potential administration route to achieve faster and higher levels of drug absorption.

It is an effective delivery system for medications, such as proteins and peptides, that are active at low concentrations and do not have little oral bioavailability. The muco-ciliary clearance mechanism's quick migration away from the absorption site in the nasal cavity is one of the causes of the low degree of peptide and protein absorption via the nasal route.

Drugs have been delivered nasally for both systemic and topical effects for a long time. Congestion, rhinitis, sinusitis, and other associated allergy or chronic disorders are all treated topically. Decongestants for symptoms of cold nasal passages, as well as antihistamines and corticosteroids for allergic rhinitis, are among the most common treatment types of medications used.

Compared to oral and intravascular methods of administration, intranasal delivery of medications is a more effective technique to ensure systemic availability. Compared to oral and parenteral delivery, it offered quicker and longer drug absorption. Analgesics (morphine), cardiovascular medications (propranolol and carvedilol), hormones (levonorgestrel, progesterone, and insulin), anti-inflammatory medications (indomethacin and ketorolac), and antiviral medications (acyclovir) are among the therapeutic groups of pharmaceuticals administered.

Advantages of nasal drug delivery

1. Drug degradation that is observed in the gastrointestinal tract is absent.
2. Hepatic first pass metabolism is avoided.
3. Rapid drug absorption and quick onset of action can be achieved.
4. The bioavailability of larger drug molecules can be improved by means of absorption enhancer or their approach.
5. The nasal bioavailability for smaller drug molecules is good.
6. Drugs that are orally not absorbed can be delivered to the systemic circulation by nasal drug delivery.
7. Studies so far carried out indicate that then as al route is an alternated parenteral route, especially, for protein and peptide drugs.
8. Convenient for the patients, especially for those on long term therapy, when compared with parenteral medication.

Limitations

1. The histological toxicity of absorption enhancers used in nasal drug delivery system is not yet clearly established.
2. Relatively inconvenient to patients when compared to oral delivery systems since there is a possibility of nasal irritation.
3. Nasal cavity provides smaller absorption surface area when compared to GIT.
4. There is a risk of local side effects and irreversible damage of the cilia on the nasal mucosa, both from the substance and from constituents added to the dosage form.
5. Certain surfactants used as chemical enhancers may disrupt and even dissolve membrane in high concentration.
6. There could be a mechanical loss of the dosage form in to the other parts of the respiratory tract like lungs because of the improper technique of administration.

Mechanism of Nasal Absorption

The initial stage of medication absorption from the nasal cavity is for the medicines to get through the mucus layer. Large, charged medications find it difficult to move through this barrier, but small, unaltered substances do so with ease. Mucin, the main protein in mucus, has a propensity to bind to solutes and obstruct diffusion. Furthermore, environmental changes (pH, temperature, etc.) may cause structural alterations in the mucus layer. Despite the fact that other absorption processes have been identified in the past, only two have been widely employed, including:

1. **First mechanism-** It involves the slow and passive water mode of transport, sometimes referred to as the paracellular pathway. The molecular weight of water-soluble compounds and intranasal absorption have an inverse log-log association. Drugs with molecular weights more than 1000 Daltons have low bioavailability.

2. **Second mechanism-** It is also referred to as the transcellular process and entails transfer via a lipoidal pathway. It is in charge of carrying lipophilic medications, whose transportation depends on how lipophilic they are. Drugs can also traverse cell membranes actively by carrier-mediated transport or by opening tight junctions. For instance, the natural biopolymer chitosan from shellfish helps drugs move through epithelial cells by opening tight junctions.

Factors Influencing Nasal Drug Absorption

The systemic bioavailability of medications delivered via nasal route is influenced by several variables. The anatomical and physiological features of the nasal cavity, the kind and features of a particular nasal medication delivery system and the physiochemical properties of the pharmaceuticals can all be impacted by these aspects. These elements are crucial for the majority of medications to achieve blood levels that are therapeutically efficacious following nasal delivery. The following is a description of the elements that affect nasal medication absorption.

1. **Physiochemical properties of drug.**
    - Molecular size.
    - Lipophilic-hydrophilic balance.
    - Enzymatic degradation in nasal cavity.
    - Stability
    - Solubility
    - Physical state of drug
    - Chemical state of drug
2. **Nasal Effect**
    - Membrane permeability.

- Environmental pH
- Muco-ciliary clearance
- Cold, rhinitis.
- Blood flow

3. **Effect of drug formulation**
   - Formulation(Concentration, pH, osmolarity)
   - Delivery effects
   - Drugs distribution and deposition.
   - Viscosity
   - Pharmaceutical excipients.

Nasal Sprays

Metered-dose pump sprays are used to administer the majority of pharmaceutical nasal preparations that are available on the market and consist of solutions, emulsions, or suspensions. Nasal sprays, often known as nasal mists, are used to administer medications directly into the nose to treat common cold or allergy symptoms such nasal congestion, or they can be used systemically (see nasal administration). The majority of nasal sprays work by using a hand-operated pump mechanism to introduce a fine mist into the nose, however delivery techniques vary. Topical decongestants, corticosteroids, and antihistamines are the three primary kinds available for local action. The actuator, the pump with valve, and the container are all part of a metered-dose pump spray system. The surface tension and viscosity of the formulation affect the metered-dose pump sprays' dosage accuracy. There are specific pump and valve combinations available on the market for solutions with greater viscosity.

Excipients Used in Nasal Spray Formulations

There are various types of excipients used in nasal formulations. Commonly used and frequently added excipients areas follows

a. **Buffers:** Nasal secretions have the potential to change the administered dose's pH, which may have an impact on the amount of unionized medication that is absorbed. Therefore, to maintain the pH in-situ, a sufficient formulation buffer capacity could be needed. Sodium citrate, citric acid, and sodium phosphate are a few examples of the buffers utilized in nasal sprays.

b. **Solubilizers:** Nasal medication administration in solution is always constrained by the drug's aqueous solubility. To increase a drug's solubility, one can employ conventional solvents or co-solvents such glycols, tiny amounts of alcohol, Transcutol (diethylene glycol monoethyl ether), medium chain glycerides, and Labrasol (saturated polyglycolyzed C8-C10 glyceride). Additional substances that can be employed include surfactants and cyclodextrins, including HP-s-Cyclodextrin, which work in conjunction with lipophilic absorption enhancers to act as a biocompatible solubilizer and stabilizer. Their effect on nasal irritancy must to be taken into account in these situations.

c. **Preservatives:** The majority of nose treatments are aqueous, thus preservatives are required to halt the growth of microorganisms. Preservatives such as parabens, benzalkonium chloride, EDTA, benzoyl alcohol, and phenyl ethyl alcohol are commonly included in nasal preparations.

d. **Antioxidants:** It could be necessary to use a tiny amount of antioxidants to stop medication oxidation. Tocopherol, sodium metabisulfite, butylated hydroxytoluene, and sodium bisulfite are examples of commonly used antioxidants. Antioxidants often don't irritate the nasal passages or alter how well drugs absorb.

e. **Humectants:** Mucous membrane crusts and drying can occur as a result of allergic reactions and chronic illnesses. Certain antioxidants and preservatives may also irritate the nose, especially when used in larger doses. Maintaining proper intranasal moisture levels is crucial to avoiding dehydration. Humectants can therefore be added, particularly to gel-based nasal treatments. Humectants do not interfere with medicine absorption and prevent nose discomfort. Sorbitol, mannitol, and glycerin are common examples.

f. **Surfactants:** By altering the permeability of nasal membranes, surfactants can be added to nasal dosage forms, potentially facilitating medication absorption through the nose. It also makes the suspension more stable. Typical instances comprise of Polysorbet.

g. **Bioadhesive polymers:** Bioadhesive polymers are compounds that can contact with biological material through interfacial forces and stay on it for extended periods of time. If the biological substance is a mucus membrane, they are also known as mucoadhesive. The type of the polymer, the pH of the surrounding medium, swelling, and physiological parameters (mucin turnover, disease status) all affect a polymer material's bioadhesive force. It is frequently advised to utilize a mix of carriers due to safety concerns regarding nose irritation.

h. **Penetration enhancer:** Chemical penetration enhancers are widely used in the nasal drug delivery.

Characterization of Nasal Spray

- pH
- Osmolality
- Viscosity
- Impurities and Degradation Products
- Preservatives and Stabilizing Excipients Assay
- Pump Delivery
- Spray Content Uniformity(SCU)
- Spray Pattern
- Droplet Size Distribution
- Particle Size Distribution

Pulmonary Routes of Drug Delivery

Introduction

Pharmaceutical companies have lately started using pulmonary drug delivery (PDD) devices to treat lung disorders that are both systemic and localized. PDD systems are recognized for their ability to easily administer the medication to the desired location within the body or to other remote locations via the bloodstream. The large surface area of alveoli in the lungs, along with their dense capillary network, make them an ideal drug-absorbing surface.

The pulmonary delivery system has been successful in treating asthma and chronic obstructive pulmonary disease (COPD) by providing symptomatic relief during the past several years due to its better efficiency and quick beginning of action. A treatment's effectiveness is mostly determined by the methods used to administer the medication and the ideal dosage range; dosages outside of these ranges may be harmful or have no therapeutic effect at all. A multidisciplinary approach to the delivery of therapeutic drugs to targets in tissues is becoming increasingly necessary, as evidenced by the sluggish development in the efficacy of treating severe illnesses.

The novel theories on immune system modulation, bio recognition, pharmacokinetics, and pharmaco dynamics regulate the efficacy of the medicine and its therapy. Often referred to as innovative or advanced drug delivery systems, these new technologies are based on multidisciplinary approaches including molecular biology, bio-conjugate chemistry, polymer science, and pharmaceutical technology. Various medication delivery and targeting systems, both established and in development, can effectively reduce drug loss and degradation, avoid negative side effects, and boost drug bioavailability. Most researchers have recognized the potential benefits of nanotechnology for more than 20 years, and these advancements have led to significant advances in medicine delivery and targeting. Novel developments in medicine delivery techniques are reducing unintended side effects and enhancing therapeutic effectiveness.

Because the lung is capable of absorbing drugs for systemic or local distribution, pulmonary delivery of drugs has gained significant scientific and biological attention in the field of health care research. The creation of fluid that lines the airways and the control of airway tone are major functions of the respiratory epithelial cells. In light of this, the pulmonary route has drawn increasing interest as a non-invasive administration method for the systemic and local delivery of therapeutic agents due to the lungs' high permeability, large absorptive surface area (adult humans' lungs have an extremely thin mucosal membrane that covers about 70–140 m2), and robust blood supply.

Advantages

1. Pulmonary drug delivery having very negligible side effects since rest of body is not exposed to drug.
2. Onset of action is very quick with pulmonary drug delivery.
3. Degradation of drug by liver is avoided in pulmonary drug delivery.
4. The ability to nebulizer viscous drug formulations for pulmonary delivery, there by overcoming drug solubility issues with the ability to use lipid, water or lipid/water emulsions as drug carriers.
5. Increased drug delivery efficacy due to size-stable aerosol droplets with reduced hygroscopic growth and evaporative shrinkage.
6. Liposomal drug formulations remain stable, when nebulizer.
7. Ability to nebulizer protein-containing solutions.
8. Inhaled drug delivery puts drug where it is needed.

Limitations

1. The orpharyngeal settlement may give local adverse effects.
2. Patients may have trouble using the delivery devices correctly.

3. Various aspects affect there producibility of drug delivery to the lungs, including physiological (respiratory scheme) and pharmaceutical (tool, formulation) variables. For the systemic delivery of drugs with a small therapeutic index, such deviations may be undesirable.
4. Drug absorption may be limited due to the barrier action of the mucus and the drug–mucus interactions.
5. Mucociliary clearance diminishes the retention time of drugs within the lungs that may affect the pharmacological efficacy of the slowly absorbed drugs.
6. The lungs are not an easily reachable surface for drug delivery, and complex delivery devices are required for targeted drug delivery.

Mechanisms of Respiratory Deposition:

- Three main processes are responsible for the deposition of inhaled aerosol particles in the respiratory tract: gravity settling, Brownian diffusion, and inertia impaction. For every breathing state, a theory is constructed to predict the dispersion and deposition of particles in the human respiratory system.
- The particle may deposit itself in various parts of the respiratory system when it enters through the mouth or nose. The airflow changes direction many times during breathing in the areas of the pharynx, larynx, nasal/mouth, and airway bifurcations.
- Particles larger than 0.5 µm have the potential to impaction deposit in these areas because to their inability to follow the air streamline. Actually, for pMDI and DPI devices, deposition by impaction in the oro-pharyngeal region still accounts for a significant amount of the dosage released.
- The primary process of inhaled particle deposition in the small airways and alveolar area is sedimentation.
- Diffusion can deposit small particles (less than 0.2 µm) in every portion of the respiratory tract. For nanoparticles smaller than 100 nm, diffusion deposition is crucial.
- When the long particle dimension is similar to the pulmonary airway diameter, intercepting the particle is crucial for elongated particles like fibrous aerosols.

Formulation of Inhalers

1. Dry powder inhalers

The purpose of the dry powder inhalers is to inhale powdered medication or excipients. Devices known as dry powder inhalers (DPIs) are used to administer an active medication in a dry powder formulation via the pulmonary route for either local or systemic effects. Bolus drug delivery devices known as dry powder inhalers are filled with solid medication that is either suspended or dissolved in a non-polar volatile propellant or in a dry powder inhaler that becomes fluidized upon inhalation by the patient. They have also been used to treat diabetes mellitus. These are frequently used to treat respiratory conditions such asthma, bronchitis, emphysema, and COPD.

The dry powder platform consists of devices that directly produce an aerosol from medication powders ranging in size from 1 to 5 µm or from mixes containing excipients. The active pharmaceutical ingredient (API) is carried by the excipients used in DPI. Lactose monohydrate is the most often used carrier.

Three phases are primarily involved in formulating DPI:

a. API Production

Particle size is a crucial criterion for API when it comes to DPI. The drug's particle size should be less than 5 µm. It need to be between two and five µm. A variety of mills are utilized to reduce drug size, but only a select number, such fluid-energy mills like the jet mill, high-peripheral-speed mills like the pin-mill, and ball mills, are suitable for DPI to reduce the size in the region of 2–5 µm.

b. Formulation of API with or without carriers.

The role of the carrier in DPI is to improve the powder's flow characteristics as well as the cohesive medicines' and fine lactose's aerosol performance. The medicine and carrier (s) are blended during the blending procedure once they have each been individually brought to the proper forms.

c. Integration of the formulation in to device

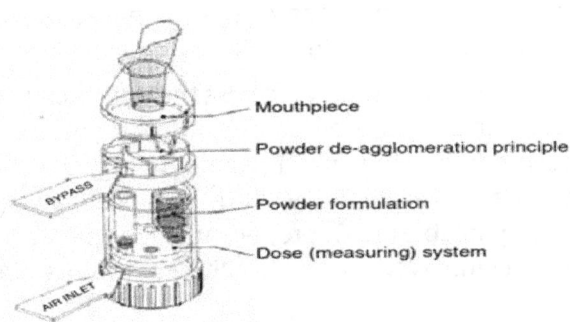

All types of devices on the market and many more in development use the same main inhaler elements. The components of the dry powder inhaler device include the mouthpiece, powder formulation, dosage metering system, and powder de-agglomeration principle.

Dry powder inhalers: Currently there are two types:

- **Unit dose devices:** A single dosage of the medication is administered using a single-unit dosing device, which is made up of individual gelatin capsules that are inserted within the device and contain a micronized drug powder and carrier system.
- **Multi dose Devices:** The factory-metered and sealed doses are packed in a way that allows the multi-unit dosage device to carry several doses without the need for reloading. Typically, the packaging consists of strips of foil-polymer blister packing, which may or may not be reloadable, or replaceable disks or cartridges.

Formulation of Pressurized Metered Dose Inhalers

With the use of a metered-dose inhaler (MDI), a patient can inhale a brief aerosolized medicine burst that contains a predetermined amount of medication. When treating respiratory conditions including asthma, chronic obstructive pulmonary disease (COPD), and others, this is the most often utilized administration method. When treating asthma and COPD, the drug in a metered dosage inhaler is often a bronchodilator, corticosteroid, or a combination of the two.

- Metered aerosols with pressure can be prepared as medication suspensions or solutions in the liquid propellant. MDIs can be made with the medication almost totally insoluble in the formulation, which is a suspension formulation, or with the medication fully dissolved in the formulation, which is a solution formulation. Solution MDIs provide a finer residual aerosol and uniform formulation (patients do not need to shake the vial just before use and sample homogeneity is not an issue) in comparison to suspension formulations.
- It is not possible to simply increase the total quantity of fine particle medication supplied by producing solution MDIs by raising the concentration of the drug. The amount of medication that may be dosed via MDIs is typically restricted since many medications are not easily soluble in HFA propellants. In the past, complexation aids or surfactants were added to MDIs to improve drug solubility in

CFC systems. Nevertheless, a large number of common excipients that are safe for human use and included in CFC formulations are soluble in the HFA system.

- The chemical stability of the medicine must be taken into consideration while choosing the technique for creating drug particles for MDI formulations. For example, proteins must be micronized with extra caution as they are heat-labile and must maintain any three-dimensional structure. In many cases, protein therapeutics are spray-dried using an additional agent (such as sodium carboxy methyl cellulose, polyvinyl alcohol, and/or polyvinylpyrrolidone (PVP)) because the three-dimensional structure and biological activity of the protein must be preserved.

- The basic requirements for formulation of MDIs are containers, propellants, and meteringvalve.

- Stuffing Metered Dose inhaler canister: propellant is liquefied at a lower temperature or higher pressure to fill the canister. In cold filling, the canister is sealed with a valve after the active substance, excipients, and propellant are cooled and filled at a temperature of around 60°C. Additional propellant is then added at the same temperature. A drug/propellant concentration is created and filled using pressure filling at almost room temperature (in fact, it's often cooled down to less than 20 degrees Celsius). Gassing is the process of adding more propellant via the valve at high pressure once the value is crimped onto the canister. The most common application of pressure filling is for inhaled aerosols.

Nebulizers

Liquids are transformed in to aerosols using a device so that they may be breathed in to the lower respiratory tract. Nebulizers are used in aerosol medication delivery to create a poly-disperse aerosol with drug particles ranging in diameter from 1 to 5 μm. While some nebulizers employ ultrasonic energy, most use compressed air for atomization. Nebulizers are often used to treat respiratory conditions such as COPD, asthma, cystic fibrosis, and others. The three primary varieties of nebulizers that are sold commercially are as follows.

- **Jet Nebulizer:** This produces an aerosol (small drug particles in the air) by compressing gas. Jet nebulizers are useful in both pediatric and adult medical settings for the acute and at-home treatment of a variety of respiratory conditions. These nebulizers needed

2–10 L/min to remove medicine from a capillary tube inside the device's reservoir. Greater varietyof particles may be produced, which would then blast against one ormore baffles to break up bigger particles into smaller ones and return them to the nebulizer in suspension.

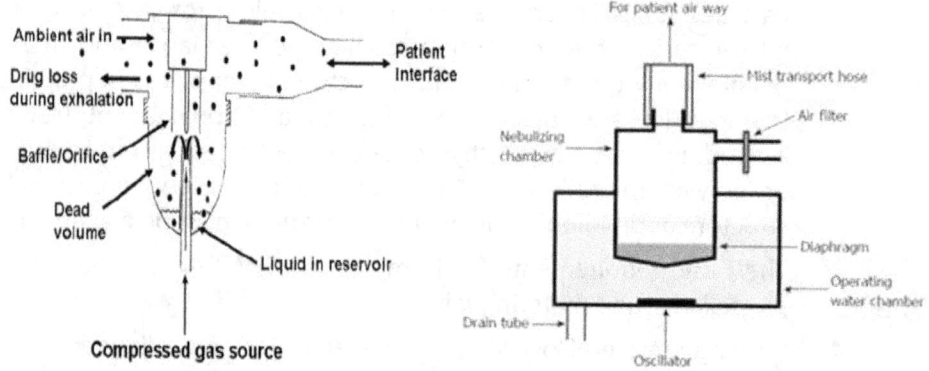

Fig: Nebulizer

- **Ultrasonic Nebulizer.** This uses high-frequency vibrations to create an aerosol. Compared to a jet nebulizer, the particles are bigger. In order to create an aerosol, ultrasonic nebulizers use a piezoelectric crystal that vibrates at high frequencies (1-3 MHz). The basis for the operation of ultrasonic nebulizers is the transducer's ability to transform electrical energy into high-frequency vibrations. We may describe these nebulizers as big volume nebulizers to provide hypertonic saline for sputum inductions because they create waves on the solution surface that are conveyed to by the vibrations the nebulizer creates.

- **Mesh Nebulizer.** Aerosol is produced when force is applied to the apertures or aperture plate found in mesh nebulizers. To create aerosol, they press liquid drugs through many holes on a mesh or aperture plate. Drug delivery using mesh and ultrasonic nebulizers was shown to be comparable in patients who were simulated to be ventilator-dependent. Mesh nebulizers can provide patients larger dosages of medication and are more effective than jet nebulizers. A few of the variables that impact mesh nebulizer efficiency include reservoir capacity, aerosol chamber size, and pore size.

Formulating Nebulizer Fluids

Nebulizer fluids are usually made with water sometimes supplemented with surfactants for suspension formulations and co-solvents such ethanol or propylene glycol. Iso-osmotic solutions with a PH of more than 5 are often used since bronchi constriction can be caused by both hypo- and hyper-osmotic solutions as well as excessive hydrogen ion concentrations. Although they may potentially induce bronchospasm, stabilizers like antioxidants and preservatives may also be used. For this reason, sulfites in particular are often avoided as antioxidants in such formulations.

Although the majority of nebulizer formulations are solutions, nebulizers can also administer medication suspensions that have been micronized. Ultrasonic nebulizers often perform badly when it comes to delivering suspensions; in contrast, jet nebulizers work better when the size of the suspended medication is reduced, releasing little to no particles when the suspended drug's droplet size is larger than the nebulizer aerosol's droplet size.

References

Aijaz A. Sheikh, subhash V. Deshmane, Kailash R. Biyani: A Text Book of Novel Drug Delivery Systems, S. Vikash and Company 2019.

Ansel HC, Popovich NG and Allen LV. Pharmaceutical dosage forms and drug delivery systems. Lea & Febiger, Philadelphia; 1990.

Aulton. M.E. Pharmaceutics; The science of dosage form design, second edition, Churchill Livingston, Harcourt publishers -2002.

Chien Y Wand Banga AK. Iontophoretic (transdermal) delivery of drugs: overview of historical development.Journal of Pharmaceutical Sciences. 1989, 78 (5); 353-354.

Jain. N.K, Controlled and novel drug delivery, first edition, CBS publishers and distributors, NewDelhi.1997.

Klausner EA, Lavy E, Friedman M, Hoffman A. Expandable gastro-retentive dosage forms. J Control Release 2003;90: 143-62.

Perkins W: Performance of PARI eFlow To the Editor.Journal of Aerosol Medicine and Pulmonary Drug Delivery 2010;23: 113-14.

Shubham Prajapati, Sanjay Saha, C. Dilip Kumar: Nebulized Drug delivery: Anoverview ,International Journal of Pharmaceutical Sciences and Research 2019; 10(8): 3575-3582.

Thorat and Santosh: Formulation and product development of nebulizer inhaler: An overview. Inc Pharmaceut Sci Res 2016; 5:30-35.

Chapter 8
Implantable Drug Delivery Systems

Introduction

Drugs can be delivered locally and specifically via implantable drug delivery devices, potentially producing therapeutic effects at lower dosages. As a consequence, they may reduce the possibility of therapeutic adverse effects while providing a chance for higher patient compliance. Because this kind of device avoids first pass metabolism and chemical degradation in the stomach and intestine, it can also increase the bioavailability of medications for which oral administration would not be appropriate.

An ideal implantable parenteral system should possess following properties:

1. **Environmental stability:** Light, air, moisture, heat, and other factors shouldn't cause implanted devices to malfunction.
2. **Biostable:** When in touch with biofluids (or medications), implantable devices shouldn't experience physicochemical degradation.
3. **Biocompatible:** Implantable devices must neither induce thrombosis or fibrosis development, nor should they trigger an immune response, since this might lead to implant rejection.
4. **Removal:** When necessary, implantable systems should be able to be removed.
5. **Non-toxic or non-carcinogenic:** Any breakdown products or additives that seep out should be totally harmless.
6. To prevent irritation, implantable devices should have a small surface area, a smooth texture, and structural traits that resemble the tissue in which they are to be implanted.
7. Drugs should be released via implanted systems for a specified amount of time at a steady pace.

Advantages and disadvantages

Advantages:
1. More effective and more prolonged action.
2. Better control over drug release
3. A significantly small dose is sufficient.

Disadvantages:
1. In vasive therapy
2. Chances of device failure
3. Limited to potent drugs
4. Biocompatibility issues

Concept of implants

Implants for drug delivery are several types:

1. Insitu forming implants(In situ depot forming systems):

a. Insitu precipitating implants

These implants are made of medication suspended in a solvent that is biocompatible. Following subcutaneous (s.c.) or intramuscular (i.m.) injection, the polymer solution precipitates polymers upon coming into contact with aqueous bodily fluids and forming implants. The purpose of in situ precipitating implants is to address certain issues related to the use of biodegradable microparticles:

1. Requirement for the reconstitution before injection
2. Inability to remove the dose one injected.
3. Relatively complicated manufacturing procedures to produce a sterile, stable and reproducible product.

b. In situ microparticle implants

This type of implants is formed to overcome the disadvantages associated with in situ Precipitating implants. These are:

1. High injection force.
2. Local irritation at the injection site.
3. Variability in the solidification rates.

4. Irregular shape of the implants formed depending on the cavity in to which the implants are introduced (implanted).
5. Undesirable high initial burst release of drugs.
6. Potential solvent toxicity.

These in situ implantable systems are comprised of an oil phase with an emulsifier and viscosity enhancer, an aqueous solution with a surfactant, and an internal phase (drug-containing polymer solution or suspension). Before being administered, the two phases are combined through a connection and kept apart in dual-chambered syringes.

2. Solid implants

Solid implants are often big bore needle injections into the s.c. or i.m. tissues, or they can be cylindrical monolithic devices implanted through a small surgical incision. Because of its ease of insertion, poor infusion, delayed medication absorption, and minimal reactivity to foreign elements, subcutaneous (s.c.) tissue is a perfect site for a device.

Drugs may be dissolved, disseminated, or imbedded in a polymer or wax/lipid matrix in these implants, which regulates the release by bioerosion, biodegradation, diffusion, or activation processes like osmosis or hydrolysis. Typically, these systems are manufactured as crushed tablets, spherical pellets, or implanted flexible/rigid molded or extruded rods. While glyceryl monostearate is a kind of wax, other polymers that are utilized include silicone, polymethacrylates, elastomers, polycaprolactones, and polylactide-co-glycolide. Typically, these implanted devices contain medications such as naltrexone and contraceptives.

3. Infusion devices

Drugs are released from infusion devices at a zero order rate by nature, and the drug reservoir can be periodically refilled. Depending on the system that powers these implanted pumps, the medications are released.

These are 3 types:
1. Osmotic pressure activated drug delivery systems
2. Vapor pressure activated drug delivery systems
3. Battery powered drug delivery systems.

Osmotic pumps

A semi-permeable membrane enclosing a drug reservoir serves as the primary design element for osmotic pumps (Fig. 8). An aperture in the membrane that permits medication release is necessary. Osmotic gradients will provide a constant fluid influx into the implant. The pressure inside the implant will rise as a result of this action, forcing the medicine to pass through the aperture. Drug release is continuous thanks to its design (zero order kinetics). A good release rate is possible with this kind of device, although drug loading is constrained.

Seminal contributions to the historical development of osmotic systems include the push-pull or GITSR system, the Rose-Nelson pump, the Higuchi-Leeper pumps, the Alzet and Osmet systems, and the elementary osmotic pump. The creation of the controlled porosity osmotic pump, asymmetric membrane-based devices, and other methods are examples of recent developments.

Osmotic agents

By providing a driving force for the absorption of water, osmotic agents are utilized in the manufacturing of the osmotic device to maintain a concentration gradient across the membrane and help to maintain medication consistency in the hydrated formulation. Ionic chemicals, such as sodium chloride, potassium chloride, magnesium sulfate, sodium sulfate, potassium sulfate, and sodium bicarbonate, are typically used as osmotic agents. Furthermore, inorganic salts of carbohydrates and sugars like sucrose, sorbitol, glucose, and others can function as potent osmotic agents.

References

Chien YW. Novel Drug Delivery Systems, 2nd Ed, New York: Marcel Dekker Inc.: NewYork,2007.

JainNK. Controlled and Novel Drug Delivery, 1 stedition, published by CBS Publishers and Distributors, NewDelhi. 1997.

Stewart SA, Domínguez-Robles J, Donnelly RF, Larrañeta E. Implantable Polymeric Drug Delivery Devices: Classification, Manufacture, Materials, and Clinical Applications. Polymers (Basel). 2018; 10(12): 1379.

Verma RK, Mishra B, Garg S. Osmotically controlled oral drug delivery. Drug DevInd Pharm. 2000;26(7):695-708.

Chapter 9
Targeted Drug Delivery

Introduction

Systemic blood circulation is used in traditional drug delivery methods, such as oral consumption or intravascular injection, to distribute the treatment throughout the body. With most therapeutic medicines, only a tiny percentage of the drug really reaches the organ or tissue that is afflicted. For example, with chemotherapy, 99 percent of the medications are not delivered to the tumor location. By delivering medicine to the targeted tissues, targeted drug delivery aims to lower the relative concentration of the medication in the target tissues.

For instance, a system can reach the desired site of action in larger quantities by eluding the host's defense mechanisms and preventing non-specific distribution in the liver and spleen. It is thought that targeted distribution would increase effectiveness while lowering negative effects.

The scientist Ehrlich originally put up the idea of tailored medications in 1906. Although it gained popularity as a theoretical idea and was discovered to be a potent substitute for efficient, site-specific therapy, the clinical use of this "magic bullet" is still difficult to achieve.

Finding the right target for a given disease state, a medication that effectively treats the condition, and an appropriate drug carrier system to deliver the medication to specific sites while avoiding immunogenic and nonspecific interactions that effectively remove foreign material from the body are the main issues that are concerning behind the success of targeted drug delivery systems.

Drug Targeting

The interaction of drug molecules with cell membrane-related biological activities at receptor sites determines a medication's therapeutic response, and this interaction is concentration dependent minimal harmful effects and maximum therapeutic index by the selective and efficient localization of the pharmacologically active moiety to the pre-identified target(s) at therapeutic concentration, while limiting its access to non-target(s) normal cellular linings.

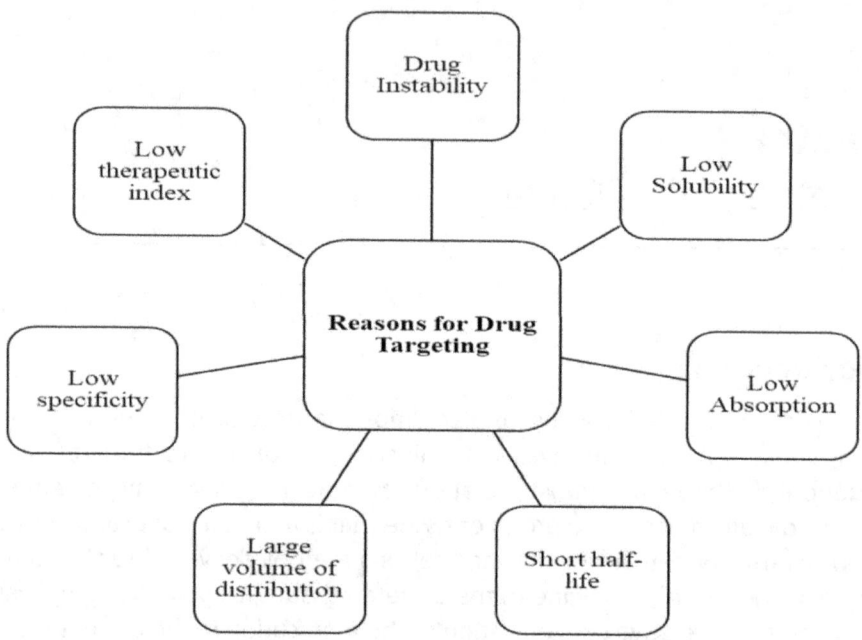

Fig. 1: *Different reason or need for Drug targeting*

Common Approaches of Targeted Drug Delivery

While there are many successful and effective drug targeting strategies, the fundamental methods for targeting a medicine to a specific location based on various study outputs may be roughly grouped into the followings.

1. Controlling the distribution of drug by incorporating it in a carrier system
2. Altering the structure of the drug at molecular level
3. Controlling the input of the drug in to bio environment to ensure a programmed and desirable bio distribution.

Properties of ideal targeted drug delivery

1. It should be nontoxic, biodegradable, biocompatible and physicochemical stable in-vivo and in-vitro
2. It should be capable to deliver the drug to target cells or tissue organ and should have uniform capillary distribution.
3. It should release the drug in a controlled and predictable manner for a suitable period of time.

4. It should efficiently maintain the drug concentration at the targeted site within the therapeutic window for prolong period of time
5. Minimal drug losses due to leakage of the carrier system should be ensured.
6. Carrier used should be biodegradable or and get readily eliminated from the body without showing any toxic interaction.
7. Its preparation should be easy or reasonably simple, reproductive and cost effective.

Important Properties Influencing Drug Targeting

The general properties influencing drug targeting can be divided into three broad categories, like properties related to Drug, Carrier and In Vivo Environment, which is briefed in below table 1.

Table1: Properties Influencing Drug Targeting

Properties related to	Important Properties/ Characteristics
Drug	Concentration, Particulate location and Distribution Molecular Weight, Physiochemical properties Drug Carrier Interaction
Carrier	Type and Amount of Excipients Surface Characteristics, Size Density
In Vivo Environment	pH, Polarity, Ionic Strength, Surface Tension, Viscosity, Temperature, Enzyme Electric Field

Strategies of Drug Targeting

a. **Passive Targeting:** Passive delivery systems are those that aim to distribute drugs into the systemic circulation. Certain colloid was a perfect substrate for passive hepatic targeting of pharmaceuticals since it could be absorbed by the Reticulo Endothelial Systems (RES), particularly in the liver and spleen.

b. **Inverse Targeting:** This kind of targeting is known as inverse targeting when efforts are under taken to prevent the passive absorption of colloidal carrier by RES. In order to accomplish inverse targeting, a significant quantity of blank colloidal carriers or macromolecules, such as dextran sulphate, are pre injected into the RES to block its usual function. This strategy results in defense mechanism suppression and RES saturation. This kind of targeting works well for directing medication onto organs other than RES.

Active targeting: Rather of relying on RES's normal absorption, this method modifies the carrier system to deliver the medicine to a specific place. One method of surface modification includes coating the surface with an albumin protein coating, a bioadhesive non-ionic surfactant, or particular cell or tissue antibodies (monoclonal antibodies).

Active targeting can be affected at different levels:

1. Limiting the distribution of the drug carrier system to the capillary bed of a pre-selected target location, organ, or tissue is known as first order targeting, also known as organ compartmentalization.
2. Second order targeting, also known as cellular targeting, is the deliberate delivery of a medication to a certain cell type, such as tumor cells, and not to healthy cells.
3. Third-order targeting, also known as intercellular organelles targeting, is the delivery of drugs to the target cells' internal organelles.

c. **Ligand-mediated Targeting:** His method uses ligands as carrier surface group(s) that may be utilized to specifically guide the carrier to the pre-designated site(s) that include the right receptor units to act as a "homing device" for the drug and carrier. The majority of carrier systems has a colloidal structure and may be precisely functionalized with a range of physiologically significant molecular legends, such as viral proteins, oligosaccharides, polypeptides, antibodies, and fusogenic residues. The ligands provide drug carriers specificity and recognition, enabling them to approach the appropriate target with selectivity and administer the medication.

Table 2: Examples of Ligands

Ligands	Target	Tumour target
Folate	Folate receptor	Over expression of folate receptor
Transferrin	Transferrin receptor	Over expression of transferrin receptor
Galactosamine	Galactosamine receptors On hepatocytes	Hepatoma

d. **Physical Targeting:** This strategy was shown to be excellent for both cytosolic delivery of genetic material or drugs that are entrapped and for targeting tumors. Changes in the pH, temperature, light intensity, electric field, and ionic strength of the environment.

Table 3: Physical Targeting Methods

Physical Targeting	Formulation System	Mechanism for Drug Delivery
Heat	Liposome	Change in Permeability
Magnetic Modulation	Magnetically Responsive Microspheres Containing Iron oxide	Magnetic Field can retard fluid Flow of particles.
Ultrasound	Polymers	Change in Permeability
Electrical Pulse	Gels	Change in Permeability
Light	Photo responsive Hydro Gels Containing Azo Derivatives	Change in Diffusion Channels, Activated by Specific Wavelength

Dual Targeting: With this targeted strategy, carrier molecules themselves have therapeutic properties of their own, which boost the medication's therapeutic impact. For instance, an antiviral medication can be loaded onto a carrier molecule that already possesses antiviral activity, and the net synergistic impact of the drug conjugate was noted.

Double Targeting: Double targeting refers to targeting a carrier system by combining temporal and geographical approaches. Targeting certain organs, tissues, cells, or even subcellular compartments with medications is known as spatial placement. The term "temporal delivery" pertains to the regulation of the drug's delivery rate to the intended location.

Combination Targeting: These targeting systems have molecularly specific carriers, polymers, and homing devices that may provide a direct path to the target location.

Advantages of drug targeting:

1. Drug administration protocols may be simplified.
2. Toxicity is reduced by delivering a drug to its target site, thereby reducing harmful systemic effects.
3. Drug can be administered in a smaller dose to produce the desire effect.
4. Avoidance of hepatic first pass metabolism.
5. Enhancement of the absorption of target molecules such as peptides and particulates.
6. Dose is less compared to conventional drug delivery system.

7. No peak and valley plasma concentration.
8. Selective targeting to infections cells that compare to normal cells.

Disadvantages of drug targeting:
1. Rapid clearance of targeted systems.
2. Immune reactions against intravenous administered carrier systems.
3. Insufficient localization of targeted systems in to tumour cells.
4. Diffusion and redistribution of released drugs.
5. Requires highly sophisticated technology for the formulation.
6. Requires skill for manufacturing storage, administration.
7. Drug deposition at the target site may produce toxicity symptoms.
8. Difficult to maintain stability of dosage form. E.g.:Resealed erythrocytes have to be Stored at 4°C.
9. Drug loading is usually law. E.g. As in micelles. Therefore it is difficult to predict/fixthe dosage regimen.

Carriers for Targeting Drugs Liposomes

Alec D. Bangham made the initial discovery of the liposome in early 1965. The name liposome is derived from the Greek word soma, which means "structure," and lipo, which means "fatty." Liposomes have a diameter ranging from several micrometers to 50 nm, making them comparatively modest in size. These are spherical vesicles with a completely phospholipid bilayer-enclosed aqueous core. Its capacity to ensnared hydrophilic and lipophilic molecules is unusual. While hydrophilic molecules may become trapped in the aqueous center, hydrophobic or lipophilic molecules are introduced into the bilayer membrane. Liposomes have gained popularity as an exploratory system and a commercial drug delivery method due to its biocompatibility, biodegradability, low toxicity, and ability to capture hydrophilic and lipophilic medicines and facilitate site-specific medication administration to cancer tissues. Liposomes have been the subject of several investigations aimed at reducing medication toxicity and/or focusing on particular cells

Advantages:
1. Suitable for delivery of hydrophobic (e.g. amphotericin B) hydrophilic (e.g. cytrabine) and amphipathic agents.
2. Liposome increases efficacy and therapeutic index of drug (actinomycin-D)

3. Liposome increase stability via encapsulation
4. Suitable for targeted drug delivery
5. Suitable to give localized action in particular tissue
6. Suitable to administer via various routes
7. Liposomes help to reduce the exposure of sensitive tissue to toxic drug.

Disadvantages:
1. Once administrated, liposome can not be removed.
2. Possibility of dumping, due to faulty administration.
3. Leakage of encapsulated drug during storage.
4. Low solubility
5. Production cost is high.

Classification

Based on structural parameters:
1. MLV: multi lamellar large vesicles .0.5µm. They have several bilayer
2. OLV: oligo lamellar vesicles 0.1-1µm. Made up of 2-10 bilayer of lipid surrounding a large internal volume.
3. UV: unilamellar vesicles (all size range)
4. SUV: small unilamellar vesicle composed of single lipid bilayer with diameter ranging from 30-70 nm
5. MUV: medium unilamellar vesicle
6. LUV: large unilamellar vesicle > 100 µm
7. GUV: giant unilamellar vesicle >1µm
8. MV: Multi vesicular vesicle >1µm

Based on method of preparation:
1. REV: single or oligo lamellar vesicles made by reverse phase evaporation method
2. MLV-REV: multilamellar vesicle made by reverse phase evaporation method
3. SPLV: stable plurilamellar vesicle
4. FATMLV: Frozen and thawed MLV
5. VET: vesicle prepared by extraction method
6. DRV: dehydration- rehydration method

Based on composition and application:
1. Conventional Liposomes (CL): Neutral or negatively charged phospholipid and cholesterol
2. Fusogenic Liposomes(RSVE): Reconstituted Sendai virus envelopes
3. pH sensitive Liposomes: Phospho lipid such as PE or DOPE with either CHEMS or OA
4. Cationic Liposomes: Cationic lipids with DOPE
5. Long Circulatory(stealth)Liposomes(LCL): Liposome that persist for prolong period of time in the blood stream
6. Immuno-Liposomes: immune liposome have specific antibody on their surface to enhance target site binding.

Preparation of Liposomes:

There are many ways of preparing liposome's. Some of the important methods are:
1. Hydration of lipids in presence of solvent
2. Ultrasonication
3. French Pressure cell
4. Solvent injection method
   a. Ether injection method
   b. Ethanol injection
5. Detergent removal Detergent can be removed by
   a. Dialysis
   b. Column chromatography
   c. Bio-beads
6. Reverse phase evaporation technique
7. High pressure extrusion
8. Miscellaneous methods
   a. Removal of Chaotropicion
   b. Freeze-Thawing

Characterisation of Liposomes:

Broadly classified in to three categories:
1. Physical characterization: evaluates parameters including size, Shape, surface features, lamellarity, phase behaviour and drug release profile.

2. Chemical characterisation: includes those studies which establish the purity, potency of various lipophilic constituents.
3. Biological characterisation: establishes the safety and suitability of formulation for therapeutic application.

Table 4: Characterisation of Liposomes

Parameters	Technique
Vesicle shape	Electron microscopy
Lamellarity	Freeze fracture electron microscopy, p-31, Nuclear magnetic resonance spectroscopy.
Vesicle size and distribution	Light microscopy, fluorescent microscopy, Electron microscopy, laserscattering photon correlation spectroscopy, gelpermeation Technique
Surface morphology and size of Vesicles	Cryo-transmission electron microscopy.
Encapsulation efficiency	Mini column centrifugation method, Protamine aggregation method
Phase response and transitional behaviour	Freeze fracture electron microscopy, Differential scanning calorimetry
Drug release	In vitro diffusion cell

Applications

Cancer chemotherapy: Liposomes are successfully used to entrap anticancer drugs. This increases circulation lifetime, protect from metabolic degradation.

Liposome as carrier of drug in oral treatment: Steroids used for arthritis can be incorporated into large MLVs.

Alteration in blood glucose levels in diabetic animals was obtained by oral administration of liposome encapsulated insulin.

Liposome for topical application: Drug like triamcinolone, methotrexate, benzocaine, corticosteroids etc. Can be successfully incorporated as topical liposome.

Liposome for pulmonary delivery: Inhalation devises like nebulizers are used to produce an aerosol of droplets containing liposome.

Niosomes

One innovative method of encapsulating a medication in a vesicular system is the use of niosomes. Niosomes get their name from the vesicle's bilayer of non-ionic surfactants. The size of the niosomes is minuscule, measured in nanometers. They are structurally similar to liposomes, yet they are superior to them in a number of ways.

Advantages of Niosomes:
a. The vesicles may act as a depot, releasing the drug in a controlled manner.
b. They are osmotically active and stable, and also they increase the stability of entrapped drug.
c. They improve the therapeutic performance of the drug molecules by delayed clearance from the circulation, protecting the drug from biological environment and restricting effects to target cells. The surfactants used are biodegradable, biocompatible and non-immunogenic.
d. They improve oral bioavailability of poorly absorbed drugs and enhance skin penetration of drugs. They can be made to reach the site of action by oral, parenteral as well as topical routes.
e. Handling and storage of surfactants requires no special conditions.
f. Due to the unique infrastructure consisting of hydrophilic, amphiphilic and lipophilic moieties together they, as a result can accommodate drug molecules with a wide range of solubilities.
g. Niosomal dispersion in an aqueous phase can be emulsified in a non-aqueous phase to regulate the delivery rate of drug and administer normal vesicle in external non-aqueous phase.

Disadvantages of niosomes:
Physical instability of the noisome vesicles is major disadvantage of the noisome drug delivery system. Aggregation: Aggregation of the noisome vesicles can be another disadvantage to be considered. Fusion: Fusion of the niosomal vesicles to form loose aggregates or to fuse into larger vesicles will affect the uniformity of the size of the noisome vesicles.
a. Leaking of entrapped drug: leakage of the entrapped drugs from the polymer system will affect the intended properties of the niosomes.
b. Hydrolysis of encapsulated drugs which limiting the shelf life of the dispersion.

Types of Niosomes

The niosomes are classified as a function of the number of bilayer (e.g. MLV, SUV) or as a function of size. (E.g. LUV, SUV) or as a function of the method of preparation (e.g. REV,DRV).

1. Multilamellar vesicles (MLV): It is made up of many bilayers that each encircles the aqueous lipid compartment in turn. These vesicles range in diameter from 0.5 to 10 μm. Among niosomes, multilamellar vesicles are the most commonly utilized. These vesicles are ideal for using as medication carriers for substances that are lipophilic.

2. Large unilamellar vesicles(LUV):These particular niosomes feature a high aqueous/lipid compartment ratio, which makes it possible to entrap higher amounts of bioactive molecules while using membrane lipids extremely little.

3. Small unilamellar vesicles (SUV): Dicetyl phosphate is added to 5(6)-carboxyfluorescein (CF) loaded Span 60 based niosomes using French press extrusion electrostatic stabilization. This process creates the majority of these tiny unilamellar vesicles from multilamellar vesicles via sonication.

Applications of Niosomes

Some of the applications of niosomes in various diseases are either proven or research are still being carried out:

Drug Targeting: The reticulo-endothelial system is the target of several medications, including niosomes. Niosome vesicles are preferentially taken up by the reticulo-endothelial system (RES). Opsonins are circulating blood factors that regulate niosome uptake. The opsonins indicate the niosome for removal. Medication localization like this is used to treat tumors in animals that have a history of spreading to the spleen and liver. Drugs localized in this way can also be utilized to treat liver parasite infections.

Drugs can also be targeted via niosomes to organs other than the RES. Since immunoglobulins adhere to the lipid surface of niosomes with ease, a carrier system (such as antibodies) can be linked to niosomes to direct them toward particular organs. Additionally, many cells have the innate capacity to identify and bind particular carbohydrate determinants; niosomes can take use of this ability to target specific cells with their carrier system.

Anti-neoplastic Treatment: The majority of antitumor medicines have serious adverse effects. Niosomes have the ability to change a drug's metabolism, increase its half-life, and increase its circulation, all of which reduce the drug's adverse effects.

In two different investigations, doxorubicin and methotrexate entrapped in niosomal beads demonstrated advantages over the un entrapped medications, including slower tumor growth and increased plasma levels with delayed clearance.

Contraceptives and delivery of targeted antibiotics.
1. Polymeric nanoparticles can be easily incorporated in to other activities related to drug delivery, such as tissue engineering.

Disadvantages:
1. Small size &large surface area can lead to particle aggregation.
2. Physical handling of nanoparticles is difficult in liquid and dry forms.
3. Limited drug loading.
4. Toxic metabolites may form. Etc.

Preparation

Nanoparticles can be prepared from a variety of materials such as polysaccharides, proteins and Synthetic polymers. Selection of matrix materials depends on many factors including:

a. Size of nanoparticles required
b. Inherent properties of the drug, e.g.stability
c. Surface characteristics such as charge and permeability
d. Degree of biodegradability, biocompatibility and toxicity
e. Drug release profile desired
f. Antigenicity of the final product.

Different techniques like polymerization, preformed polymers or ionic gelation etc are used.

Preparation of nanoparticles from dispersion of preformed polymer:

Dispersion of drug in preformed polymers is a common technique used to prepare biodegradable nanoparticles from poly (lactic acid) (PLA), poly (D, L-glycolide) (PLG), poly(D,L-lactide-co-glycolide)(PLGA).These can be accomplished by different methods described below.

a. Solvent evaporation
b. Nano precipitation
c. Emulsification/solvent diffusion
d. Salting out
e. Dialysis
f. Supercritical fluid technology(SCF)

Preparation of nanoparticles from polymerization of monomers
a. Emulsion
b. Mini emulsion
c. Microemulsion
d. Interfacial polymerization
e. Controlled/Living radical polymerization

Ionic gelation or coacervation of hydrophilic polymers

Table: Techniques for Physicochemical Characterization of Nanoparticles

Parameters	Technique
Particle size and morphology	Transmission electronic microscopy, scanning (electron,-force,tunneling)microscopy, freeze-fracture electron microscopy, photon correlation spectroscopy
Drug content in vitro drug release	Ultra centrifugation followed by quantitative analysis of in vitro release characteristics under physiologic and sink conditions.
Molecular weight crystallinity	Gel permeation chromatography, X-ray diffraction, Differential scanning calorimetry
Surface charge Surface hydrophobicity	Zeta potential measurement, hydrophobic interaction chromatography, contact angle measurement
Surface chemical analysis	Secondary ion mass spectrometry, X-ray photo electron spectroscopy, nuclear magnetic resonance, Fourier Transform Infrared spectroscopy
Protein adsorption	Two-dimensional polyacrylamide gel electrophoresis

Application of Nano Particulate Drug Delivery Systems:
- Vaccine adjuvant.
- Ocular delivery.
- Internalization: Internalization within mammalian cells can be achieved by surface functionalized carbon nanotubes.

- Vaccine delivery: Conjugation with peptides may be used as vaccine delivery structures
- Gene delivery: with the advancement in molecular dynamics simulations, the flow of water molecules through surface-functionalized carbon nanotubes has been modelled in such a way so that they can be conveniently utilized as small molecule transporters in transporting DNA, indicating potential use as a gene delivery tool.
- Transport of peptides, nucleic acids and other drug molecules Incorporation of carboxylic or ammonium groups to carbon nanotubes enhances their solubility which makes them more suitable for the transport of peptides, nucleic acids and other drug molecules.
- Reduced toxicity and increases the efficacy.
- Cancer therapy: This technology is being evaluated for cancer therapy. Nano shells are tuned to absorb infrared rays when exposed from a source outside the body and get heated and cause destruction of the tissue. This has been studied in both in vitro and in vivo experiments on various cell lines.
- Diagnosticpurposes: They are useful for diagnostic purposes in whole blood immunoassays E.g. Coupling of gold nano shells to antibodies to detect immunoglobulins in plasma and whole blood. etc.

Monoclonal Antibodies

The immune system employs antibodies, which are proteins, to recognize and destroy foreign substances like bacteria and viruses. Every antibody identifies a particular antigen that is particular to its target. Antibodies are a great tool for identifying and measuring a wide range of targets, including medicines, serum proteins, and microbes, due to their high specificity. Antibodies may precipitate soluble antigens, agglutinate (clump) cells, opsonize and kill bacteria with complement, and neutralize medications, poisons, and viruses using in-vitro testing.

Monoclonal antibodies (mAB) are generated by B-cell clones of a single parent or a single hybridoma cell line. They are a single kind of identical immunoglobulin that are directed against a particular epitope (antigen, antigenic determinant). One B-cell lymphocyte and one myeloma cell combine to generate a hybridoma cell line. Certain myeloma cells spontaneously produce single mAB antibodies. Monclonal antibodies vary from polyclonal antibodies in that they are derived from a single B-cell clone and then target a single epitope. Antibodies that are produced from several cell lines are called polyclonal antibodies. Their amino acid sequences are different.

History and Development

- Paul Enrlich at the beginning of 20thcentury coined the term "magic bullets" and postulated that, if a compound could be made that selectively targets a disease-causing organism, then a toxin for that organism could be delivered along with the agent of selectivity.
- In the 1970s, the B-cell cancer multiple myeloma was known. It was understood that these cancerous B-cells all produce a single type of antibody (a para protein).
- In 1975, Kohler and Milstein provided the most outstanding proof of the clonal selection theory by fusion of normal and malignant cells (Hybridoma technology) for which they received Nobel Prize in 1984.

Advantages of Monoclonal antibodies

a. Though expensive, monoclonal antibodies are cheaper to develop than conventional drugs because it is based on tested technology.
b. Side effects can be treated and reduced by using mice-human hybrid cells or by using fractions of antibodies.
c. They bind to specific diseased or damaged cells needing treatment.
d. They treat a wide range of conditions.

Disadvantages of Monoclonal antibodies:

a. Time consuming project- anywhere between 6-9 months.
b. Very expensive and needs considerable effort to produce them.
c. Small peptide and fragment antigens may not be good antigens- monoclonal antibody may not recognize the original antigen.
d. Hybridoma culture may be subject to contamination.
e. System is only well developed for limited animal and not for other animals.
f. More than 99% of the cells do not survive during the fusion process– reducing the range of useful antibodies that can be produced against an antigen
g. It is possibility of generating immunogenicity.

Application of Monoclonal antibodies

1. Diagnostic Applications:

Monoclonal antibodies have revolutionized the laboratory diagnosis of various diseases. For this purpose, MAbs may be employed as diagnostic reagents for biochemical analysis or as tools for diagnostic imaging of diseases.

(A) MAbs in Biochemical Analysis:

In the laboratory, enzyme-linked immunosorbent assays (ELISA) and radioimmunoassays (RIA) frequently employ diagnostic procedures based on the use of MAbs as reagents. These assays quantify the levels of various tissue and cell products (blood group antigens, blood clotting factors, interferons, interleukins, histocompatibility antigens, tumor markers) as well as hormones (insulin, human chorionic gonadotropin, growth hormone, progesterone, thyroxine, triiodothyronine, thyroid stimulating hormone, gastrin, renin). Many MAb-based diagnostic kits have entered the commercial market in recent years. For example, early identification of the following illnesses and ailments is now feasible.

Pregnancy:
Pregnancy by detecting the urinary levels of human chorionic gonadotropin
Cancers:
Prostate specific antigen is used to estimate prostate cancer while plasma carcino embryonic antigen is used to estimate colorectal cancer. The prognosis of malignancies benefits from tumor marker estimate in addition to diagnosis. That is, after therapy, a progressive decline in a particular tumor marker is seen along with shrinkage of the tumor.

Hormonal disorders: Thyroid stimulating hormone, triiodothyronine, and thyroxine are analyzed for thyroid diseases under hormonal disorders.

Diseases caused by infections: Infections by measuring the quantities of antigens in the blood that are unique to the infectious agent, such as the herpes simplex virus and Neisseria gonorrhoea antigens for the diagnosis of sexually transmitted infections.

(A) MAbs in Diagnostic Imaging:

Immunoscintigraphy is the term for the diagnostic imaging method that uses radio labeled—MAbs to image illnesses. The radioisotopes technetium (99) and iodine (131) are frequently used to mark MAb. The patients get intravenous injections of the radioisotope-tagged MAb.

Through radioactive imaging, these MAbs may be localized to specific areas, such as tumors. Single photon emission computed tomography (SPECT) cameras have been employed recently to provide a more sensitive three-dimensional representation of the locations where radiolabeled MAbs have localized.

When it comes to diagnostic tools, immunoscintigraphy outperforms CT, ultrasound, and magnetic resonance imaging. For example, because radiolabeled MAbs are tumor specific, immunoscintigraphy can distinguish between malignant and non-cancerous development. Other imaging methods cannot accomplish this. Monoclonal antibodies have proven to be effective in the diagnostic imaging of bacterial infections, malignancies, and cardiovascular illnesses.

2. Therapeutic Applications:

A. Cardiovascular diseases: Myocardial infarction:

Anywhere there is myocardial necrosis, or the loss of heart cells, the cardiac protein myosin is visible. Myosin and, thus, the location of myocardial infarction are detected using antimyosin MAb that has been radioisotope-labeled with indium chloride (111 In). After intravenous injection, radio labeled MAb is typically imaged 24-48 hours later.

Either a conventional gamma camera or single photon emission computed tomography (SPECT) is used for this. Radiolabeled antimyosin MAb can be used to determine the extent and location of cardiac injury. For this reason, this method is helpful in the diagnosis of heart attacks.

B. Deep vein thrombosis(DVT):

1. The term DVT describes the development of thrombus, or blood clots, in the blood vessels, usually in the lower limbs. Antibodies labeled with radioisotopes specific for fibrin or platelets can be used to diagnose deep vein thrombosis (DVT). Usually, the imaging is completed four hours following the injection. Fibrin specific
2. MAbs are successfully used for the detection of clots in thigh, pelvis, calf and knee regions.
3. Atherosclerosis is the term used to describe the thickening and loss of flexibility of artery walls. Peripheral and coronary artery disorders are brought on by atherosclerotic plaques. Heart disease development has been linked to atherosclerosis. Using an imaging method, atherosclerotic lesions may be identified using MAb labeled with a radiolabel aimed against active platelets

References

Andrew MS, James PA, Jedd DW. Mono clonal Antibodies in Cancer Therapy, Cancer Immunity, 2012; 12:14 –21

Archana S, Jinjun S, Suresh G, Alexander RV, Nagesh K, Omid CF. Nano particles for Targeted and Temporally Controlled Drug Delivery, Multi functional Nano particles for Drug Delivery Applications: Imaging, Targeting, and Delivery, Nano struct. Sci. Technol. 2012; 9 – 29.

Bhargav E, Madhuri N, Ramesh K, Anand manne, Ravi V. Targeted Drug Delivery-AReview,World J. Pharm. Pharm.Sci. 2013;3(1):150 -169

Gupta M, Sharma V. Targeted drug delivery system: A Review, Res. J. Chem. Sci.2011;1(2):135 – 138

Jaya A, Shubhini S,Anubha K. Targeting : New Potential Carriers for Targeted DrugDeliverySystem,Int. J.Pharm.Sci. Rev. Res.2011;8(2):117-123

LachmanL, Lieberman HA, KanigJL. The Theory and Practice of Industrial Pharmacy. In Roop Khar, Vyas SP, Farhan A, Jain Gaurav, editors. Novel Drug Delivery Systems, 3rded, Varghese Publishing House; 2014. p. 872-906

LachmanL, Lieberman HA, KanigJL.The Theory and Practice of Industrial Pharmacy. In Roop Khar, Vyas SP, Farhan A, Jain Gaurav, editors. Targeted Drug Delivery Systems, 3rd ed, Varghese Publishing House;2014. p. 907-43

Lasic DD, Application sof Liposomes. In Lipowsky R, Sackmann E, editors. Volume1,2014.p. 493-94.

Nurit B, Itai B. Antibody-Based Immun otoxins for the Treatment of Cancer, Antibodies, 2012; 1:39–69

Panchagnula R, Dey CS. Monoclonal Antibodies in Drug Targeting, J. Clin. Pharm. Ther.1997; 22:7–19

Theresa M, Allen. Ligand-Targeted Therapeutics in Anticancer Therapy, Nature 2002;2: 750 – 763

Chapter 10
Ocular Drug Delivery System

Introduction

The novel approach in which drug can instill on the cull de sac cavity of eye is known as ODDS. Specifically sterile preparations of dosage forms intended for topical application, intraocular administration, per ocular administration, or usage in conjunction with an ophthalmic device are known as ophthalmic preparations. The dose forms that are most frequently used include ointments, suspensions, and solutions. Precorneal loss factors, such as solution drainage, lacrimation, tear dynamics, tear dilution, tear turnover, conjunctival absorption, nonproductive absorption, transient residence time in the cul-de-sac, and the relative impermeability of the corneal epithelial membrane, are the main causes of poor bioavailability of drugs from ocular dosage forms. Numerous approaches for ocular medication administration are taken into consideration; they range from simple formulation methods to increasing drug availability. The most common forms of ODDS preparations include gels, ointments, ocular inserts, microspheres, and nanoparticles.

Advantages of ODD

1. It increases accurate dosing.
2. It provides sustained and controlled drug delivery system.
3. It increases the ocular bioavailability of drug by increasing the corneal contact time.

Disadvantages of ODDS

1. Dosage form cannot be terminated during emergency.
2. It Interfere with vision.
3. It is difficult tin placement and removal.

Anatomy of eye

The outer sclera, middle choroid layer, and inner retina make up the wall of the spherical structure that is the eye. The inner layers are protected by the thick fibrous covering known as the sclera. With the exception of the cornea, which is transparent and lets light into the eye, it is white. Numerous blood veins may be seen in the choroid layer, which is located inside the sclera and is transformed into the colored iris at the front of the eye. The location of the biconvex lens is just behind the pupil. Eighty percent of the eye ball is made up of vitreous humor, a viscous material that fills the chamber behind the lens. Aqueous humor fills the anterior and posterior chambers, which are located between the cornea, iris, and lens, respectively. A back of the eye is light detecting retina.

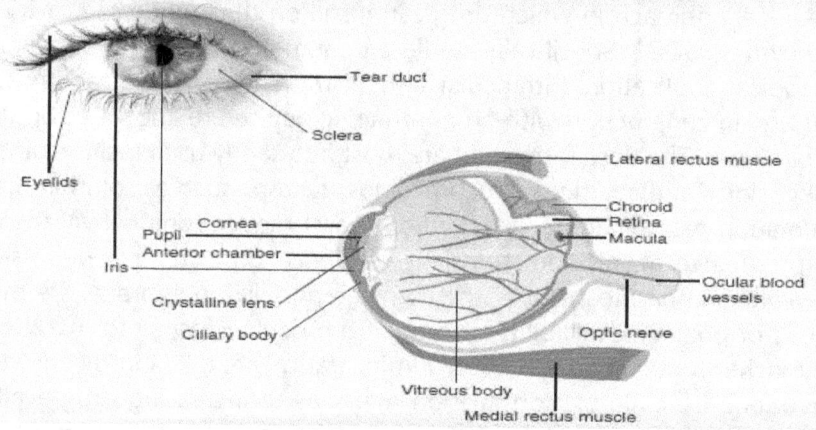

Fig. 1: Anatomy of eye Intra ocular barriers

1. **Tear:** Tear film, the pre corneal barrier, lowers the effective concentration of medications administered because of drug molecule binding to tear proteins, faster clearance, and dilution by tear turnover (1μl/min). The dosing volume of instillation is generally 20–50 μl whereas the size of cul-de-sac is only 7–10 μl. The excess volume may spill out on the cheek or exit through the naso lacrimalduct.

2. **Cornea:** The stroma, endothelium, and epithelium make up the three layers of the cornea, together with a mechanical barrier that prevents the entry of foreign materials into the eye. Every layer has a unique polarity and a structure that limits the pace at which drugs can permeate it. Because of its lipophilic nature, the corneal epithelium forms tight connections that prevent paracellular drugs from penetrating the tear film. The fibrils of collagen make up the stroma. Lipophilic medication molecules are unable to penetrate the stroma's highly hydrated

structure. The innermost monolayer of hexagon-shaped cells, the corneal endothelium serves as a barrier dividing the stroma from the aqueous humor. Because of their leakiness, endothelial connections allow macromolecules to move easily between the stroma and aqueous humor.

3. **Conjunctiva**: The thin, transparent membrane known as the conjunctiva, which covers the globe and eyelids, aids in the creation and upkeep of the tear film. There are many capillaries and lymphatics in the conjunctiva or episclera. As a result, medications applied to the conjunctiva may be eliminated via lymph and blood. Because the conjunctival blood vessels lack a strong junction barrier, drugs can enter the bloodstream by convective transport via the vascular endothelium layer's paracellular holes and pinocytosis.

4. **Sclera**: The sclera mainly consists of collagen fibres and proteoglycans embeddedin an extracellularmatrix.The molecular radius determines scleral permeability, which falls down approximately exponentially with molecular radius. The human sclera is somewhat thick around the limbus (0.53 ± 0.14 mm), thin at the equator (0.39 ± 0.17 mm), and significantly thicker near the optic nerve (0.9-1.0 mm). The posterior sclera is made up of a looser weave of collagen fibers than the anterior sclera. The rise in hydrophobic/lipophilic medicines indicates a decrease in sclera permeability. Drugs that are hydrophilic may diffuse more readily than those that are lipophilic via the aqueous medium of proteoglycans in fiber matrix pores. The medication molecule's charge may have an impact on how easily it passes through the sclera. Because positively charged medications attach to the negatively charged proteoglycan matrix, they may have poor permeability.

5. **Choroid/Bruch'smembrane**: One of the body's most highly vascularized tissues, the choroid supplies blood to the retina. In humans, the fenestrated choroidal capillary endothelial cells have a diameter of 20–40 μm. As people age, Bruch's membrane (BM) thickens. Increased calcification of elastic fibers, increased collagen fiber cross-linking, and greater turnover of glycosaminoglycans are the results of these modifications. In BM, lipofuscin and advanced glycation end products build up. Changes in choroid and BM thickness may have an impact on the permeability of drugs from the subconjunctival space into the retina and vitreous.

6. **Retina**: The internal limiting membrane (ILM) is one of the barriers preventing drugs from penetrating from the vitreous to the retina.

The retina and vitreous are separated by the ILM, which is made up of ten different extracellular matrix proteins. There are two ways that drugs can enter the retinal pigment epithelium (RPE): transcellular and paracellular. Small molecules can move out of the subretinal spaces via active transport via the transcellular pathway or by paracellular inter-RPE cellular clefts, propelled by the forces of hydrostatic and osmotic pressures.

7. **Blood-Retinal Barrier**: Medication transfer from blood into the retina is limited by the blood retinal barrier (BRB).The tight connections between RPE and retinal capillary endothelial cells, known as oBRB for the outer BRB and iBRB for the inner BRB, make up the BRB. Muller cells and astrocytes assist the action of iBRB. There are insufficient vesicles and no windows in the retinal capillary endothelial cells. Endocytosis or transcytosis, which may be receptor-mediated or fluid phase needing adenosine triphosphate, is described as the function of these endothelial vesicles. Under normal circumstances, Muller cells sustain neuronal activity and ensure that iBRB functions properly. As a result, oBRB (RPE) limits the ability of medications to enter the retina from the choroid. Between the choroid and the sensory retina lies the RPE, a monolayer of highly specialized hexagon-shaped cells. The RPE's tight connections effectively prevent intercellular penetration of the sensitive retina.

Methods to overcome barriers

1. Physical methods

Physical force-based methods, initially utilized in transdermal drug delivery, generally require a power driven physical device to deliver energy to the barriers, thereby enhancing transient drug transport.

1. Iontophoresis

   It is the procedure via which ions are injected into tissues or cells by direct current. Drug distribution across biological membranes is improved by iontophoresis, which is the application of a low-intensity electrical current that causes the drug molecule to electrorepel and electro-osmose. Electro-osmosis can improve the transport of both neutral and charged molecules by convective solvent flow, whereas electrorepulsion only pertains to the mobility of ionic medications. The drug's size, charge, and charge to molecule weight ratio, among other physicochemical factors, and the biological membrane's electrical characteristics determine the relative contributions of electrorepulsion and electro-osmosis. Ocular iontophoresis is a quick, painless, safe method of drug delivery that often results in the delivery of a high concentration of medication to a particular location.

2. Sonophoresis/Ultrasound

To enhance medicationtransport across biological membranes, including ocular barriers, a sound field greater than 20 kHz is used. The non-thermal (such as cavitation, acoustic streaming, and mechanical stress) and thermal effects with ultrasound parameters,co-administration of microbubbles, and drug properties are all taken into consideration in the processes for ultrasound enhanced drug delivery, since these factors all affect the effectiveness of the drug's delivery. Cavitation, which is defined as the development of microbubbles as a result of an acoustic pressure differential inside the coupling medium, is typically regarded as the primary reason for increased drug delivery. At low ultrasonic intensities, stable cavitation often results in enhanced corneal permeability; however, at greater ultrasound strengths, both stable and inertial cavitations play significant roles.

3. Microneedles

Microneedles (MLs) are needles or arrays of needles that are sized at micrometers and are created using customizing micro electronics instruments. Drugs can pass through biological membranes when MLs are applied because they can form small transport channels. Numerous ML fabrication approaches have been utilized, resulting in a variety of shapes, sizes, materials andconfigurations. Insertion of MLs across the corneal epithelium can result in enhanced medication delivery into the cornea and anterior portion of the eye. A wide range of polymeric MLs have proven particularly beneficial for intrascleral medication administration. Ocular MLsmay be divided into four varieties based on how they are delivered: solid microneedles, drug-coated microneedles, dissolving microneedles,and hollow microneedles.

2. Chemical approaches

An established method in therapeutic drug delivery is the chemical alteration of pharmaceuticals to increase their physicochemical qualities, such as stability, permeability, solubility, and evasion of the efflux pump, as well as their therapeutic efficacy. Chemically modified medications with a predictable metabolic bioconversion in the eye can be used because of the metabolic activity of ocular tissues.

The most important strategies in chemical approaches for ocular delivery are

- Designing ocular drugs that are inactive at sites other than the eye (prodrugs)
- Designing drugs that undergo sequential metabolic conversion and finally reach the target(retro metabolic design)
- Chemical modification of a known inactive metabolite or analog to restore the rapeutic activity that transforms back into the in active meta bolite in apredictable one-step bio transformation (SD)

Ocular formulations

1. Drug delivery systems to anterior segment of the eye
2. Drug delivery systems to posterior segment of the eye
3. Advanced delivery system
4. Vesicular drug delivery system

Drug delivery systems to anterior segment of the eye

Eye-Drops

Drugs that operate on the surface of the eye or in the eye are frequently supplied as solutions, emulsions, or suspensions. Since this drug delivery mechanism does not reach acceptable drug concentrations in the posterior tissues, eye drops are often employed for anterior segment problems. Retention of a solution in the eye can be affected by a number of characteristics of eye drops, including viscosity, osmolality, concentration of hydrogen ions, and injected volume.

Opthalmic Inserts

Sterile preparations having a solid or semisolid consistency, specifically formulated for ocular use, are called ophthalmic inserts. The lower fornix is where the inserts are inserted, whereas the upper fornix or corneas are used less frequently.

Classification of ocular inserts

Based upon their solubility behaviour

1. Insolubleinserts
2. Solubleinserts
3. Bioerodibleinserts

1. Insoluble ocuserts

Insoluble ocuserts can be classified into two categories such as reservoir system and matrixsystem.

A. Reservoir system

The medication is released in this system either by an osmotic mechanism or by diffusion. It comprises liquid, gel, colloid, semisolid, solid matrix, or drug-containing carrier, in that order.

Diffusional insertor ocuserts

This innovative ocular medicine delivery device is based on porous membrane occuserts. Diffusional release mechanisms underpin the drug release from occusert implants. The medicine is allowed to diffuse through the core reservoir of the diffusional systems at a carefully controlled pace thanks to specially engineered semipermeable or microporous membranes around it. The lacrimal fluid that passes through the membrane in such a device regulates the release of the medication until an internal pressure is achieved that forces the drug out of the reservoir. Diffusion through the membrane, which one may regulate, governs the pace of medication delivery. Diffusion through the membrane, which one may regulate, governs the pace of medication delivery. For instance, pilocarpine, an ocular hypotensive medication, has a uniform regulated release (20 or 40µg/hr) for seven days with the ocusert device. It is composed of an inner layer of pilocarpine in alginate gel with di(ethylhexyl) phthalate as a release enhancer, sandwiched between two outside layers of ethylene vinyl acetate co polymer (EVA).

Ocusert has certain demerits such as difficult to inserting the device, ejection of device from eye and irritation during insertion.

Osmotic inserts

The osmotic inserts are usually composed of a central part bounded by a peripheral part and are of two types:

Type1

The main component consists of a single drug reservoir encircled by discrete tiny deposits of polymer, either with or without an extra osmotic solute scattered over a polymeric matrix. The second peripheral component of these inserts was an insoluble semipermeable polymer sheet. The polymer matrix ruptures as a result of the osmotic pressure acting on it, creating perforations. The medication is then discharged from the deposits through these pores close to the device's surface.

Type2

There are two distinct sections in the center. The drug and osmotic solutes are separated into two compartments; the osmotic solute reservoir is surrounded by a semi-permeable membrane, while the drug reservoir is covered by an elastic impermeable membrane. This kind's second peripheral component resembles type 1's. Through the semipermeable polymeric barrier, the tear fluid diffuses into the peripheral deposits, wetting them and causing them to dissolve. The hydrostatic pressure created by the solubilized deposits pushes on the polymer matrix, rupturing it into apertures. The drug is subsequently delivered by the only hydrostatic pressure through these pores from the deposits close to the device's surface, which is against the eye.

B. Matrix systems

A certain class of insoluble optical devices and contact lenses comprise the majority of the second category matrix system. The three-dimensional network or matrix it is made of covalently cross-linked hydrophilic or hydrophobic polymers can hold water, an aqueous drug solution, or solid components.

Contact lenses

The first line of treatment for vision correction is contact lenses. These structures are formed and composed of hydrophilic or hydrophobic polymers that are cross-linked covalently to produce a three-dimensional network or matrix that may hold solid, aqueous, or water-based components. When a hydrophilic contact lens is soaked in a drug solution, it absorbs the drug, but does not give a delivery as precise as that provided by other non-soluble ophthalmic systems. The drug release from such a system is generally very fast at the beginning and then declines exponentially with time. The release rate can be decreased by incorporating the homogenous mixture of drug during the manufacture or by adding a hydrophobic component. Contact lenses are divided into 5 parts such as rigid, semi-rigid, elastomeric, soft hydrophilic and bio-polymeric

2. Soluble Ophthalmic inserts

Soluble inserts correspond to the oldest class of ophthalmic inserts. Soluble inserts normally defined as erodible, monolithic polymeric devices that releasing the drug and do not need removal while undergo gradual dissolution. Through polymer swelling true dissolution occurs mainly, while to a chemical or enzymatic hydrolytic process erosion corresponds. In swelling- controlled devices in a glassy polymer, the active agent is homogeneously dispersed. Water from the tear fluid begins to penetrate the matrix when the insert is placed in the eye, then by releasing their drug content, swelling and consequently polymer chain relaxation and drug diffusion take place.

Types of soluble ophthalmic inserts
a. Based on natural polymers e.g. collagen.
b. Based on synthetic or semi synthetic polymers

A. Natural polymers
Collagen is the preferred natural polymer utilized in the production of soluble ophthalmic inserts. Before applying the therapeutic agent to the eye, it is best to soak the insert in a drug-containing solution, dry it off, and then rehydrate it. The amount of binding agent used, the concentration of the drug solution the composite is soaked in, and the length of the soaking process will all affect how much drug is loaded. The medication is progressively released from the spaces between the collagen molecules as the collagen degrades.

B. Synthetic and semi-synthetic polymer
This is predicated on the usage of polymers, namely synthetic polymers like polyvinyl alcohol and semi-synthetic polymers like cellulose derivatives. Reduced release rate can be achieved by utilizing Eudragit, a polymer often used for enteric coating or as the insert's coating agent. One hydrophobic polymer that can be utilized to reduce the deformation of the insert and avoid impaired vision is ethylene cellulose.

3. Bio-erodible ocular inserts
Bio-erodible polymers (e.g., polyester derivatives, cross-linked gelatin derivatives) dissolve these inserts by the hydrolysis of chemical bonds. The ability to adjust the rate of erosion of these bio-erodible polymers by altering their final structure during synthesis and adding cationic or anionic surfactants is a tremendous benefit. A few significant ocular inserts that are either commercially available (SODI) or in advanced stages of development (Mindisc, Ocufit, and collagen shields).

Soluble ophthal micdrug insert
Soviet scientists created the soluble ophthalmic drug insert (SODI), a tiny oval wafer, for cosmonauts who were unable to utilize eye drops while in weightlessness. A soluble copolymer of ethyl acrylate, acrylamide, and N-vinyl pyrrolidone is called a SODI. It comes in the shape of oval-shaped, sterile thin film or wafers that weigh between 15 and 16 mg. next its insertion into the upper conjunctival sac, the SODI softens in 10 to 15 seconds, taking on the shape of

the eyeball; the film then transforms into a polymeric clot in the next 10 to 15 minutes, which eventually dissolves in 1 hour while releasing the medication.

Collagen shields

Over twenty-five percent of the protein in animals' bodies is made up of collagen, which is the structural protein of skin, tendons, ligaments, and bones. Nowadays, collagen shields made of bovine corium (dermis) or porcine scleral tissue are used in collagen shield manufacturing. Type I and some type III collagen are present in these materials. They have a contact lens-like shape and are delivered dried, so you have to rehydrate them before inserting them. The amount of time a lens takes to dissolve is determined by variations in the collagen crosslinking caused by ultraviolet radiation (UV) during production. There are now three types of collagen shields that dissolve in 12, 24, and 72 hours. The dimensions of corneal collagen shields are 14.5–16.0 mm in diameter, 9 mm for the base curve, and 0.15–0.19 mm in the center.

Ocufit

The 1992-patent Ocufit is a silicone elastomer sustained release rod device being developed by Escalon Ophthalmics Inc. (Skillman, NJ). Its dimensions and form were intended to match those of the human conjunctival fornix. As a result, its diameter and length are limited to 1.9 mm and 25–30 mm, respectively; nevertheless, lesser versions are intended for toddlers and newborns.

The Minidis cocular therapeutic system

The Minidisc ocular therapeutic system (OTS), a monolytic polymeric device first reported by Bawa et al. (Bausch and Lomb, Rochester, New York), is shaped like a tiny (4-5 mm) contact lens, with a convex and a concave face, the latter of which roughly conforms to the sclera of the eye. According to reports, the device's specific dimensions and form make it simple to position beneath either the top or lower lid without sacrificing comfort, visibility, or oxygen permeability. Table 1 lists the ocular insert devices.

Table 1: Ocular inserts devices

Name	Description
Soluble ocular drugInsert	Small oval wafer, composed of soluble co polymers consisting of actylamide, N-venyl pyrrolid onean dethylacetate, soften on insertion
New ophthalmic drug delivery system	Medicated solid poly vinyl alcohol flag that is attached to a paper-covered-with handle. On application, the flag detaches and gradually dissolves, Releasing the drugs

Collagen shields	Erodible disc consist of cross-link porcines cleralcollagen
Ocusert	Flat, flexible elliptical insoluble device consisting of two layers, enclosing a reservoir, use commercially to deliver Pilocarpine for 7days
Minidisc orocular therapeutic	system 4-5 mm diameter contoured either hydro philicor hydrophobic disc
Lacrisert	Rose-shape device made from Hydroxy propyl cellulose use for the eye Syndrome as an alternative to tears
Gelfoam	Slabs of Gel foam impregnated with a mixture of drug and cetylester wax in Chloroform
Drydrops	A preservative free of hydro philicpolymer solution that is freeze dried on the tip of a soft hydrophobic carrier strip, immediately hydrate in tear strip

Punctal Plugs

To prolong the retention time and increase absorption and efficacy after instillation of eye drops, inhibition of drainage through nasola crimal system using punctual plug into the panctaisa long standing approach. Efficacy of an ocular hypotensive agent in eye drops in conjuction with punctual occlusion by punctual plug is reported.

Sub conjunctival/ Episcleral Implants

Biodegradable polymers and medications can be used to create a scleral plug, which can be inserted into the pars plana area of the eye and delivers medication dosages gradually over several months as it breaks down. The kind of polymers utilized, their molecular weights, and the amount of medication in the plug all affect the release profiles. The silicone matrix episcleral implant LX201 (Lux Biosciences, USA) is intended to provide cyclosporine A to the surface of the eye for a duration of one year. The implant has a rounded top in touch with the anterior surface and a flat bottom in contact with the episclera.

Ointment and Gels

With ophthalmic ointments and gels, the duration of medication interaction with the external eye surface can be extended. Gels and ointments can thereby increase the duration of effect and improve the ocular bioavailability of medications. The ointment fragments into tiny droplets and stays in the cul de sac for a long time as a drug depot. However, matting of the eyelids and blurring of vision can restrict their uses.

Drug delivery systems to posterior segment of the eye

1. Intravitreal Implants

Durasert™TechnologySystem

The Durasert TM technology system (pSivida Crop.,US) distributes medications for predefined durations ranging from days to years by utilizing a drug core surrounded by one or more polymer layers. The polymer layers' permeability regulates the drug's release. Cytomegalo virus retinitis can be treated with ganciclovir-loaded implants using the DurasertTM technology system. This implant, which is composed of PVA and ethylene vinyl acetate copolymer (EVA), releases ganciclovir over the course of six to eight months by passive diffusion through a tiny hole in the EVA at the base of the device.

Novadur™Technology

The FDA has authorized Ozurdex® (Allergan Inc., US), an intravitreal implant made of PLGA (6.5 mm in length and 0.45 mm in diameter) and contains 0.7 mg of dexamethasone.It is used to treat macular edema brought on by central and branch retinal vein occlusions (BRVO and CRVO). Ozurdex® is injected into the vitreous cavity using a specialized injector equipped with a 22 gauge needle.

I-vation™TA

The vitreous of the eye is treated with triamcinolone acetonide (TA) administered using vationTM technology (Sur Modics Inc., US). The titanium helical coil (0.5 mm in length and 0.21 mm in width) used in the I-vationTM intravitral implant is coated with TA (925 μg), non-biodegradable polymers (methyl methacrylate), and EVA.This implant has a minimum two-year in vivo lifespan.

NT-501

Via an implanted device in the vitreous, encapsulated cell technology (Neurotech Pharmaceuticals Inc., US) delivers ciliary neutropic factor (CNTF) extracellularly through long-term, sustained intraocular release at consistent levels. It contains human RPE cells that have undergone genetic modification to produce human CNTF recombinant. The device is made up of six strands of cell-loaded polyethylene terephthalate yarn encased in a sealed, semi-permeable membrane capsule. A tiny sclera incision is used to surgically implant the device into the vitreous, and one end of the device is secured with a single stitch through a titanium loop. The semipermeable barrier shields the contents from host cells immunologic attack while permitting the outward diffusion of CNTF and other cellular metabolites and the inward diffusion of nutrients required to ensure the cell survival in the vitreous cavity.

2. Injectable particulate systems

IBI-20089

Icon Bioscience Inc.'s VerisomeTM drug delivery platform technology is used in IBI-20089 to deliver triamcinolone acetonide (TA).In contact with saline, the IBI-20089 solution takes on a milky, slightly opaque hue and gels.IBI-20089 is a biodegradable benzyl benzoate solution containing TA.It is intended to administer medication with a single intravitreal injection for up to a year.

RETAAC

Patients with diabetic macular edema (DME) may benefit from intravitreal injections of RETAAC, which have been shown to be more effective than injections of bare TA. For a year, eyes treated with RETAAC demonstrated reduced retinal thickness and enhanced visual acuity.The retina is safe and tolerant to it.

Cortiject®

Target tissue activated corticosteroid prodrug is encapsulated in an oily carrier and phospholipid surfactant in Cortiject® (Novagali Pharma S.A.), a preservative-free emulsion.

Visudyne®

Photosensitizer is a component of the intravenous liposomal formulation Visudyne® (QLT Ophthalmics Inc., USA).Verteporfin in photodynamic therapy for pathologic myopia, suspected ocular histoplasmosis, or AMD-related subfoveal choroidal neovascularization.Low density lipoprotein (LDL), a type of plasma lipoprotein, has been demonstrated to increase the number of LDL receptors on tumor cells, which may improve the transport of hydrophobic verteprofin to malignant tissue.Since phosphatidyl glycerol makes up a significant portion of the Visudyne® formulation, undissociated verteporfin that is still encapsulated in liposomes is accumulated in vascular endothelial cells via LDL receptor-mediated endocytosis. Verteporfin released in blood from liposomes is associated with LDL and uptakes in neovascular tissues.

Advanced delivery system

1. Cellen capsulation

Encapsulated cell technology (ECT) is the process of entrapping immunologically isolated cells with hollow fibers or microcapsules prior to their delivery into the eye.It makes it possible to deliver therapeutic proteins to the posterior areas of the eye in a regulated, continuous, and long-term manner. The vitreous humour of the patient's eye secretes ciliary neutrophic factor due to the polymer implant that contains genetically engineered human RPE cells. Chronic ocular illnesses such as neuroprotection in glaucoma, antiangiogenesis in choroidal neovascularization, and anti-inflammatory agents in uveitis are treated with ECT.

2. Gene therapy

Gene therapy techniques are employed in conjunction with tissue engineering to treat blindness caused by corneal disorders, cataracts, glaucoma, etc. Gene transfer and gene therapy applications involve the manipulation of many viruses, including as adenovirus, retrovirus, adeno-associated virus, and herpes simplex virus. Ocular gene transfer through topical application is the fastest method. Because of their high efficacy, retroviral vectors are used, which limits their clinical usage. The utilization of improved delivery systems extends the duration of the vector's interaction with the ocular surface, potentially improving transgene expression and facilitating non-invasive administration.

3. Stemcell Therapy

The cornea and retina, which are essential for visual function, can be restored with cell therapy. Currently, treating eye diseases involves either getting rid of the harmful substance or trying to lessen its effects. The limbal stem cells are used the most successful ocular application transplanted from a source other than the patient for the renewal of corneal epithelium. The sources of limbal cells include donors, autografts, cadavereyes and cellsgrownin culture.

4. Protein and peptide therapy

A key component of medication delivery is the transportation of therapeutic proteins and peptides to the eye. However, a number of constraints, including solubility, metabolism, size, and membrane permeability, limit how effectively they may be delivered. Hydrophilic peptides with low membrane permeability can have their permeability increased by structurally altering the molecule. The preferred method for systemic distribution of such big molecules is not the ocular route. Through the transscleral pathway, immunoglobulin G is successfully supplied to the retina with negligible systemic absorption.

5. Scleral plug therapy

Made of biodegradable polymers and medications, scleral plugs can be placed at the pars plana region of the eye by a straightforward operation. When it biodegrades, effective dosages of medications are released for several months. The type of polymers utilized, their molecular weight, and the amount of medication in the plug all affect the release profiles. The plugs are useful in the treatment of vitreoretinal illnesses that need virectomy, proliferative vitreoretinopathy, and CMV retinitis that reacts to recurrent intravitreal injections.

6. siRNA therapy

The choroidal neovascularization is treated with siRNA therapy. These strategies are applied in clinical studies, where the siRNA is targeted against either VEGF or VEGF receptor 1 (VEGFR1). Topical use of siRNA is intended to inhibit corneal neovascularization by targeting VEGF or its receptors. Gene delivery in ocular disease processes also occurs via siRNA treatment. According to reports, siRNA may be used in the pathophysiology and creation of novel therapeutics for ocular illnesses, drawing on both in vitro and in vivo research. Using polymer vesicles or liposomes linked with antibodies, new encapsulated siRNA are created.

7. Oligonucliotide therapy

The idea behind oligonucleotide (ON) therapy is to prevent the production of cellular proteins by interfering with the translation of mRNA into proteins or the transcription of DNA into mRNA. The anti sense molecules prevent the creation of proteins and interfere with gene expression.

Antisense oligonucliotide effectiveness is found to be influenced by several factors. The length of the ON species is the main factor to take into account. It has been suggested that ON lengths between 17 and 25 bases are ideal since longer ONs may partially hybridize with non-target RNA species. The main obstacle to taking into account while delivering RNA and DNA oligonucleotides to cells is biological stability. It is possible to prevent nuclease activity by altering bases, sugar moieties, and phosphate backbones.

8. Aptamer

Oligonucleotide ligands known as aptamers are employed to bind molecules with a high degree of affinity. Through an iterative process of adsorption, recovery, and reamplification, it is separated from synthesized nucleic acid. It exhibits great selectivity and very low binding with the target compounds. The RNA aptamer pegaptanib sodium (Pfizer) targets the VEGF isoform that is mainly in charge of vascular permeability and pathological eye neovascularization.

9. Ribozyme therapy

RNA enzymes, also known as ribozymes, are single-stranded RNA molecules with the ability to adopt three-dimensional conformations and catalyze the cleavage, ligation, and polymerization of nucleotides involving DNA or RNA at particular sites. By cleaving the phosphodiester backbone at a particular cutting location, it attaches itself to the target RNA molecule and renders it inactive. In cases of autosomal dominant retinitis pigmentosa (ADRP), ribozyme administration appears to be beneficial for managing the condition. Gene mutations causing altered proteins that cause photoreceptor cells to undergo apoptosis are the cause of ADRP.

Vesicular system

1. Liposomes

Liposomes are lipid-based vesicles that have an aqueous volume inside of them. Liposomal drug delivery systems are capable of delivering lipophilic medications to the ocular system. They are in close proximity to the surfaces of the cornea and conjunctiva, which is advantageous for poorly absorbed, low-partition-coefficient, and poorly soluble medicines. Thus, it improves the absorption of drugs into the eyes.

2. Noisome

Niosomes are nonionic surfactant vesicles that have potential applications in the delivery of hydro phobic or amphi philic drugs. They are more stable than liposomes. Hence they can target drug to eye very easily.

3. Pharmacosomes

Pharmacosomes are a useful technique for achieving targeted medication delivery and controlled release, among other desired therapeutic objectives. Any medication having an active hydrogen atom (-COOH, -OH, -NH2, etc.) can be esterified to a lipid with or without a spacer chain, producing a molecule that is highly amphiphilic and that will help the organism move its membranes, tissues, or cell walls. These are described as colloidal dispersions of pharmaceuticals that are covalently bonded to lipids. Depending on the chemical nature of the drug-lipid combination, these can exist as ultrafine vesicular, micellar, or hexagonal aggregates. The pharmacosomes exhibit improved stability, easier corneal transport, and a regulated release profile.

References

Agrawal YK. Current status and advanced approaches in ocular drug delivery system. J. Glob. Tren. in Phar. Sci, 2011; 2(2):131-148.

Barar J, Javadzadeh AR, Omidi Y. Ocular novel drug delivery: impacts of membranes and barriers: Expert Opin. Drug Deliv. 2008; 5(5): 567-581.

Chien YW, Ed. Novel drug delivery systems, Vol-50, Inform a healthcare, USA, 2011; 269-275.

Geroski, D.H.; Edelhauser, H.F. Drug delivery for posterior segment eye disease. Invest. Ophthalmol.Vis. Sci.2000; 41:961-964.

Jeffery D. Henderer and christopher J. Rapuano., In: Laurence L. Bruton Johns. La. Kerth L. parker (eds.),Good man and Gilman`s the pharmacological basis of Therapeutics, Mc Garw-Hill, Newyork, 2006; 1707-1735.

Lee, S.S.; Hughes, P.M.; Robinson, M.R. Recent advances in drug delivery systems for treating ocular complications of systemic diseases. Curr. Opin. Ophthalmol. 2009; 20:511-519.

Menqi SA and Desh Pande SG (Eds.), In: N.K. Jain, Controlled and Novel drug delivery systems, CBS publishers,New delhi, 2004;82-96.

Singh K, Novel Approaches in Formulation and Drug Delivery using Contact Lenses. J. Bas.Clin. Phar,2011; 2(2): 87-101.

Singh V. The challenges of ophthalmic drug delivery: a review, Int. J. Drug. Disc, 2011; 3(1):56-62.

Sudhakar M, Sahoo CK, Bhanja S, Rao SRM, Panigrahi B. Concepts and Principles of Modified Release Drug Delivery System.Vol.1; first edition, Starline Publishing House, Bhubaneswar, Odisha.2019.

Thakur RR. Modern Delivery Systems for Ocular Drug Formulations: A Comparative Overview W.R.T Conventional Dosage Form. Int. J . Res. In. Phar & Biomed Sci, 2011; 2 (1): 8-18.

Vyas SP, Khar RK, Ed. Targeted and controlled drug delivery, CBS Publishers, New delhi, 2011;374-375.

Wilson CG, Zhu YP, KurmalaP, RaoLS, Dhillon B. Opthamic drug Delivery. In: Anya M. Hillery, Andrew W. Lloyd James Swabrick (eds.), Drug Delivery and targeting, Taylor and Francise-library, London, 2005;298-318.

Chapter 11
Intrauterine Drug Delivery System

Introduction to Intrauterine Drug Delivery System

Intrauterine drug delivery systems (IUDs) represent a sophisticated approach to delivering therapeutic agents directly to the uterus, harnessing the unique environment of the female reproductive system for targeted drug administration. These devices, often made of biocompatible materials, are inserted into the uterus where they gradually release medications over an extended period. This method offers several advantages over conventional drug delivery routes, including improved efficacy, reduced side effects, and enhanced patient compliance.

Intra-uterine drug delivery systems was to compile the recent literature with special focus on various Intra-uterine approaches that have recently become leading methodologies in the field of site specific orally administered controlled release drug delivery. The drug releases in uterine to terminate the pregranacy. Advantages and Disadvantages of IUDDS covered in details. In intrauterine drug delivery system IUD (Intauterine Devices) are used and which are of various types and which are effective for three to ten years depending on type. The IUD is a long-acting reversible method of contraception. An intra-uterine device is a special device that fits inside of the uterus. Intrauterine Device (IUD) is a small object that is inserted through the cervix and placed in the uterus to prevent pregnancy. A small string hangs down from the IUD into the upper part of the vagina. The IUD is not noticeable during intercourse. IUDs can last 1-10 years. They affect the movements of eggs and sperm to prevent fertilization. They also change the lining of the uterus and prevent implantation. IUDs are 99.2-99.9% effective as birth control. They do not protect against sexually transmitted infections, including HIV/AIDS. Insertion of an IUD takes only about 5 to 10 minutes. A clinician must insert an IUD. It is usually done when you are on your period. The clinician will perform a pelvic exam and check to see where your uterus is positioned. They will then insert a speculum into your vagina to see your cervix and then wash your cervix with an antiseptic solution. An IUD prevents pregnancy by stopping sperm from reaching an egg that your ovaries have released. It does this by not letting sperm go into the egg. The IUD will be inserted up through the opening of your cervix into your uterus. It is put inside using a special applicator that keeps the IUD flat and closed until it is at the top of your uterus.

Definition and Overview: An intrauterine drug delivery system refers to a medical device designed to deliver drugs or therapeutic agents directly into the uterine cavity for local or systemic effects. These systems typically consist of a small, flexible device inserted into the uterus, where it releases controlled doses of medication over a specified period. Unlike oral medications or injections, which can lead to systemic side effects or require frequent dosing, IUDs provide sustained release of drugs at the target site, optimizing therapeutic outcomes while minimizing systemic exposure.

Historical Background: The concept of intrauterine drug delivery dates back centuries, with early attempts involving the use of natural materials such as plant extracts or medicated pessaries. However, modern IUDs evolved from the development of intrauterine devices (IUDs) for contraception in the mid-20th century. The first hormonal IUD, containing levonorgestrel, was introduced in the 1990s, paving the way for the integration of drug delivery technology into contraceptive devices. Since then, ongoing research and innovation have expanded the applications of IUDs to include hormone therapy, treatment of gynecological disorders, and prevention of endometrial diseases.

Importance and Applications: Intrauterine drug delivery systems play a crucial role in women's health by offering targeted treatment options for various reproductive health conditions. These systems are particularly valuable in contraception, providing long-acting, reversible birth control options that offer high efficacy and convenience. Hormonal IUDs, in particular, have gained popularity for their ability to provide continuous, low-dose hormone therapy while minimizing systemic side effects. Additionally, IUDs are utilized in the management of gynecological disorders such as menorrhagia, endometriosis, and adenomyosis, offering localized treatment and symptom relief. The versatility and efficacy of intrauterine drug delivery systems make them a promising approach in the field of women's health, with ongoing research focused on expanding their applications and improving patient outcomes. Hormonal IUDs (referred to as intrauterine systems in the UK) work by releasing a small amount of levonorgestrel, a progestin. Each type varies in size, amount of levonorgestrel released, and duration. The primary mechanism of action is making the inside of the uterus uninhabitable for sperm. They can also thin the endometrial lining and potentially impair implantation but this is not their usual function. Because they thin the endometrial lining, they can also reduce or even prevent menstrual bleeding. As a result, they are used to treat menorrhagia (heavy menses), once pathologic causes of menorrhagia (such as uterine polyps) have been ruled out.

Anatomy and Physiology of the Female Reproductive System

The female reproductive system is a complex network of organs and hormones responsible for the production of gametes, fertilization, pregnancy, and childbirth. Understanding the anatomy and physiology of this system is essential for comprehending the mechanisms underlying intrauterine drug delivery.

Structure of the Uterus: The uterus, also known as the womb, is a pear-shaped organ located in the pelvis between the bladder and the rectum. It consists of three main layers:

Endometrium: The innermost layer of the uterus, the endometrium, is composed of glandular epithelium and stroma. It undergoes cyclic changes in response to hormonal fluctuations during the menstrual cycle, thickening to prepare for implantation of a fertilized egg and shedding during menstruation if pregnancy does not occur.

Myometrium: The middle layer, the myometrium, is comprised of smooth muscle tissue responsible for the rhythmic contractions that facilitate childbirth. These contractions are regulated by hormonal signals and neural input.

Perimetrium: The outermost layer, the perimetrium, consists of a serous membrane that covers the surface of the uterus and helps to anchor it within the pelvic cavity.

Hormonal Regulation of the Menstrual Cycle: The menstrual cycle is regulated by hormones. Luteinizing hormone and follicle-stimulating hormone, which are produced by the pituitary gland, promote ovulation and stimulate the ovaries to produce estrogen and progesterone.

The menstrual cycle is regulated by the complex interaction of hormones:

Luteinizing hormone, follicle-stimulating hormone, and the female sex hormones estrogen and progesterone.

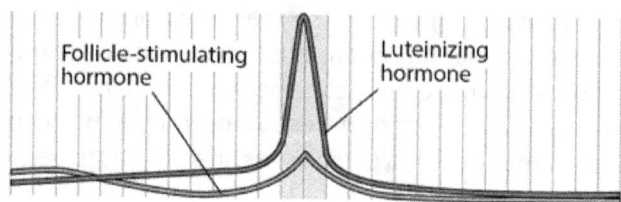

Pituitary Hormone Cycle

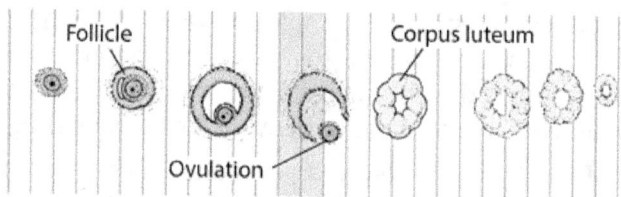

Ovarian Cycle

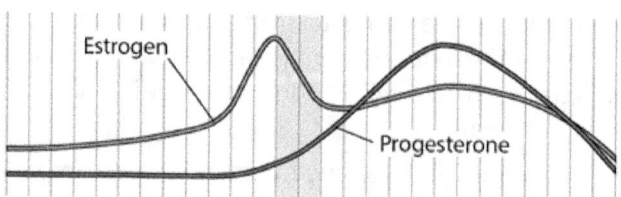

Sex Hormone Cycle

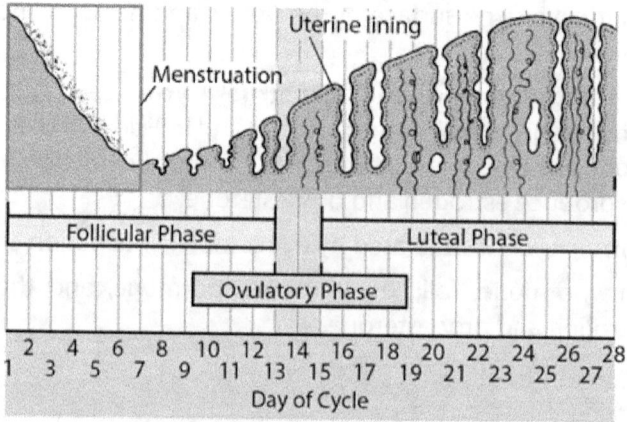

Endometrial Cycle

The menstrual cycle has three phases:
- Follicular (before release of the egg)
- Ovulatory (egg release)
- Luteal (after egg release)

The menstrual cycle begins with menstrual bleeding (menstruation), which marks the first day of the follicular phase.

When the follicular phase begins, levels of estrogen and progesterone are low. As a result, the top layers of the thickened lining of the uterus (endometrium) break down and are shed, and menstrual bleeding occurs. About this time, the follicle-stimulating hormone level increases slightly, stimulating the development of several follicles in the ovaries. (Follicles are sacs filled with fluid.) Each follicle contains an egg. Later in this phase, as the follicle-stimulating hormone level decreases, usually only one follicle continues to develop. This follicle produces estrogen. Estrogen levels increase steadily.

1. **Menstrual Phase:** The menstrual cycle begins with menstruation, marked by the shedding of the endometrial lining. Estrogen and progesterone levels are low during this phase, leading to vasoconstriction and subsequent shedding of the endometrium.

2. **Follicular Phase:** Following menstruation, the follicular phase begins with the maturation of ovarian follicles under the influence of follicle-stimulating hormone (FSH) secreted by the pituitary gland. As the follicles develop, they produce increasing amounts of estrogen, which stimulates the proliferation and thickening of the endometrium in preparation for implantation.

3. **Ovulation:** Midway through the menstrual cycle, typically around day 14 in a 28-day cycle, a surge in luteinizing hormone (LH) triggers ovulation, the release of a mature egg from the ovary. This surge is preceded by a rapid increase in estrogen levels, which promotes the release of LH from the pituitary gland.

4. **Luteal Phase:** Following ovulation, the ruptured follicle transforms into a structure called the corpus luteum, which secretes progesterone. Progesterone, along with estrogen, maintains the thickened endometrial lining in preparation for implantation and pregnancy. If fertilization does not occur, the corpus luteum degenerates, leading to a decline in estrogen and progesterone levels and the onset of menstruation.

Factors Affecting Drug Absorption in the Uterus

Drug absorption in the uterus is influenced by various factors, including the physicochemical properties of the drug, the characteristics of the delivery system, and the physiological environment of the uterus. Key factors affecting drug absorption include:

Blood Supply: The uterus is highly vascularized, with extensive blood flow to support its reproductive functions. Drugs delivered to the uterus may be rapidly absorbed into the bloodstream, leading to systemic effects.

Endometrial Permeability: The permeability of the endometrial epithelium can vary depending on factors such as menstrual cycle phase, hormonal fluctuations, and the presence of inflammation or infection. Drugs must penetrate the endometrial barrier to reach target tissues or exert their pharmacological effects.

Drug Formulation: The formulation of the drug delivery system, including its size, shape, composition, and release kinetics, can significantly impact drug absorption in the uterus. Optimizing these parameters is essential for achieving desired therapeutic outcomes while minimizing side effects.

The pH of the uterine environment and the solubility of the drug can influence its absorption and distribution within the uterus. Drugs that are poorly soluble or unstable under acidic conditions may require formulation strategies to enhance their bioavailability and efficacy.

This detailed examination provides a comprehensive understanding of the anatomy and physiology of the female reproductive system, including the structure of the uterus, hormonal regulation of the menstrual cycle, and factors influencing drug absorption in the uterus. These insights are crucial for designing effective intrauterine drug delivery systems and optimizing their therapeutic potential in women's health care.

Types of Intrauterine Drug Delivery Systems

Intrauterine drug delivery systems (IUDs) encompass a diverse array of devices designed to deliver therapeutic agents directly into the uterus for local or systemic effects. These systems can be broadly classified into two main categories: non-hormonal IUDs and hormonal IUDs. Each type offers unique advantages and applications, with distinct mechanisms of action governing their pharmacological effects.

Non-Hormonal IUDs

Non-hormonal IUDs, also known as inert IUDs or copper IUDs, are contraceptive devices that do not contain any hormones. Instead, they are typically made of plastic or a combination of plastic and metal, with a copper component added to enhance contraceptive efficacy. Copper IUDs work primarily by creating a hostile environment for sperm, impairing their motility and viability, and preventing fertilization. Additionally, copper ions released by the device may alter the composition of cervical mucus, inhibiting sperm penetration into the uterus. One of the most widely used non-hormonal IUDs is the copper-containing intrauterine device (Cu-IUD), such as the ParaGard® T 380A. This device consists of a T-shaped plastic frame wrapped with copper wire and is inserted into the uterus by a healthcare provider. Cu-IUDs provide long-term contraception, with a typical duration of effectiveness ranging from 5 to 10 years depending on the specific product.

Hormonal IUDs

Hormonal IUDs, also known as levonorgestrel-releasing IUDs, are contraceptive devices that release a progestin hormone, typically levonorgestrel, directly into the uterine cavity. These devices are designed to provide long-acting, reversible contraception while minimizing systemic side effects associated with traditional hormonal contraceptives. Hormonal IUDs work by thickening cervical mucus, inhibiting sperm motility, and thinning the endometrial lining, thereby reducing the likelihood of implantation. One of the most widely used hormonal IUDs is the levonorgestrel-releasing intrauterine system (LNG-IUS), such as Mirena®, Skyla®, and Liletta®. These devices consist of a T-shaped frame containing a reservoir of levonorgestrel hormone, which is released gradually over several years. LNG-IUSs offer highly effective contraception, with typical durations of effectiveness ranging from 3 to 7 years depending on the specific product.

Mechanism of Action

The mechanisms of action of non-hormonal and hormonal IUDs differ significantly, reflecting their distinct compositions and modes of contraceptive action.

Non-Hormonal IUDs

The primary mechanism of action of non-hormonal IUDs, such as copper IUDs, involves the release of copper ions into the uterine cavity. Copper ions have spermicidal properties, inhibiting sperm motility and viability, and preventing fertilization. Additionally, copper ions may alter the biochemical composition of cervical mucus, making it less conducive to sperm penetration.

Hormonal IUDs

Hormonal IUDs, on the other hand, release a progestin hormone, typically levonorgestrel, directly into the uterine cavity. Levonorgestrel thickens cervical mucus, reducing sperm penetration, and inhibits sperm motility, impairing their ability to reach and fertilize the egg. Furthermore, levonorgestrel thins the endometrial lining, making it less hospitable for implantation, thereby providing an additional mechanism of contraceptive efficacy. A comprehensive overview of the types of intrauterine drug delivery systems, including non-hormonal IUDs, hormonal IUDs, and their mechanisms of action. By understanding the differences between these devices, healthcare providers can make informed decisions regarding contraceptive options for their patients, optimizing efficacy and patient satisfaction.

Design and Development of Intrauterine Drug Delivery Systems

Designing and developing effective intrauterine drug delivery systems (IUDs) requires careful consideration of various factors, including materials selection, manufacturing techniques, and formulation considerations. This chapter explores the key aspects involved in the design and development process, highlighting the importance of each component in achieving optimal drug delivery outcomes.

Materials Selection: The choice of materials plays a critical role in the performance, biocompatibility, and safety of intrauterine drug delivery systems. Ideal materials should possess several key characteristics, including biocompatibility, mechanical strength, stability, and compatibility with the drug formulation. Common materials used in the fabrication of IUDs include:

Polymeric Materials: Biocompatible polymers such as polyethylene, polyurethane, and silicone are frequently used in the construction of IUDs due to their flexibility, inertness, and ease of processing. These materials can be tailored to achieve specific drug release kinetics and mechanical properties, making them suitable for a wide range of applications.

Metals: Some IUDs incorporate metal components, such as copper or stainless steel, to enhance contraceptive efficacy or provide structural support. Copper IUDs, for example, utilize copper wire wound around a plastic frame to release copper ions into the uterine cavity, while stainless steel may be used to reinforce the device and ensure proper placement within the uterus.

Drug-Loaded Polymers: In certain cases, drugs or therapeutic agents may be directly incorporated into polymeric matrices or coatings to achieve sustained release and localized delivery. Drug-loaded polymers offer precise control over drug release kinetics and can be tailored to meet specific therapeutic requirements.

Manufacturing Techniques: The manufacturing process plays a crucial role in the quality, consistency, and scalability of intrauterine drug delivery systems. Various techniques may be employed to fabricate IUDs, depending on the desired design, materials, and drug delivery requirements. Common manufacturing techniques include:

Injection Molding: Injection molding is a widely used manufacturing technique for producing polymer-based IUDs. This process involves injecting molten polymer into a mold cavity under high pressure, where it solidifies to form the desired shape and structure of the device. Injection molding offers precise control over dimensions, geometry, and surface features, making it suitable for mass production of IUDs with complex designs.

Extrusion: Extrusion is another common manufacturing technique used to fabricate polymer-based IUDs. In this process, molten polymer is forced through a die to form continuous shapes or profiles. Extrusion allows for the production of IUD components such as rods, tubes, or filaments with uniform cross-sectional dimensions and mechanical properties.

Coating and Encapsulation: For drug-loaded IUDs, coating and encapsulation techniques may be employed to incorporate drugs into polymeric matrices or coatings. This may involve methods such as solvent casting, spray coating, or electrospinning to achieve uniform drug distribution and controlled release profiles.

Formulation Considerations: Formulation considerations are critical in optimizing the performance, stability, and bioavailability of drug-loaded intrauterine drug delivery systems. Several factors must be taken into account during the formulation process, including:

Drug Solubility and Stability: The solubility and stability of the drug in the delivery system are key determinants of drug release kinetics and efficacy. Formulation strategies such as selection of appropriate excipients, pH adjustment, and use of stabilizing agents may be employed to enhance drug solubility and stability.

Drug Release Kinetics: The desired release profile of the drug, whether immediate, sustained, or controlled, must be carefully considered during formulation. Factors such as polymer composition, drug loading, and device geometry can influence drug release kinetics and duration of action.

Biocompatibility and Safety: Formulations used in intrauterine drug delivery systems must be biocompatible and non-toxic to ensure patient safety. Materials and excipients should be thoroughly evaluated for potential adverse effects, including irritation, inflammation, or allergic reactions.

The design and development of intrauterine drug delivery systems, covering materials selection, manufacturing techniques, and formulation considerations. By carefully considering these factors, researchers and developers can design IUDs that offer optimal drug delivery performance, biocompatibility, and therapeutic efficacy.

Pharmacokinetics and Pharmacodynamics of Intrauterine Drug Delivery

Intrauterine drug delivery systems (IUDs) offer a unique approach to delivering therapeutic agents directly to the uterus, influencing both pharmacokinetic and pharmacodynamic processes. Understanding the intricate interplay between drug absorption, distribution, metabolism, and excretion (ADME), as well as drug release kinetics, therapeutic efficacy, and safety profiles, is essential for optimizing the performance of IUDs in clinical practice.

Absorption, Distribution, Metabolism, and Excretion (ADME): The pharmacokinetics of drugs delivered via intrauterine drug delivery systems are governed by processes of absorption, distribution, metabolism, and excretion within the female reproductive system.

Absorption: Following insertion into the uterine cavity, drugs released from IUDs may be absorbed through the endometrium and enter the systemic circulation. Absorption rates and extent depend on various factors, including the physicochemical properties of the drug, the formulation of the delivery system, and the characteristics of the uterine environment.

Distribution: Once absorbed, drugs may distribute within the uterus, exerting local effects on target tissues and cells. Distribution within the systemic circulation may also occur, leading to distribution to other organs and tissues throughout the body.

Metabolism: Metabolic processes may occur within the uterus or in other organs, leading to the biotransformation of drugs into metabolites. Metabolism may influence the pharmacological activity, duration of action, and elimination of drugs delivered via IUDs.

Excretion: Drugs and their metabolites may be eliminated from the body through various routes, including renal excretion, biliary excretion, and metabolism. The extent and rate of excretion depend on factors such as drug clearance, renal function, and hepatic metabolism.

Drug Release Kinetics: The release kinetics of drugs from intrauterine drug delivery systems play a crucial role in determining the onset, duration, and intensity of pharmacological effects. Drug release kinetics are influenced by factors such as the composition and design of the delivery system, the solubility and diffusivity of the drug, and environmental conditions within the uterine cavity.

Zero-Order Release: Some IUDs are designed to release drugs at a constant rate over time, resulting in zero-order release kinetics. This sustained release profile ensures a steady concentration of the drug within the uterus, maintaining therapeutic levels over an extended period.

First-Order Release: Other IUDs may exhibit first-order release kinetics, where drug release rates decrease exponentially over time. This may result in initial burst release followed by gradual decline, influencing the duration and intensity of pharmacological effects.

Therapeutic Efficacy and Safety Profiles: The therapeutic efficacy and safety profiles of intrauterine drug delivery systems are influenced by various factors, including drug pharmacodynamics, patient characteristics, and device design. Evaluating these parameters is essential for assessing the clinical utility and potential risks associated with IUDs.

Efficacy: The efficacy of IUDs depends on their ability to deliver therapeutic agents to target tissues and cells within the uterus, achieving desired pharmacological effects. Factors such as drug release kinetics, dose, and duration of action influence the therapeutic efficacy of IUDs in preventing pregnancy, managing gynecological disorders, or providing hormone therapy.

Safety: Safety considerations include the risk of adverse effects, local tissue reactions, and systemic toxicity associated with the use of intrauterine drug delivery systems. Biocompatibility, stability, and compatibility with the uterine environment are critical factors in ensuring the safety of IUDs and minimizing the potential for harm to patients.

The pharmacokinetics and pharmacodynamics of intrauterine drug delivery systems, covering processes of ADME, drug release kinetics, therapeutic efficacy, and safety profiles. By understanding these principles, healthcare providers can optimize the design and utilization of IUDs to maximize therapeutic benefits while minimizing risks to patients.

Clinical Applications and Therapeutic Uses

Intrauterine drug delivery systems (IUDs) offer versatile and effective solutions for a wide range of clinical applications in women's health. From contraception to the treatment of gynecological disorders and the management of reproductive health conditions, IUDs play a crucial role in improving patient outcomes and quality of life.

Contraception: Intrauterine drug delivery systems are widely used as highly effective contraceptive methods, offering long-acting, reversible birth control options for women of reproductive age. Both non-hormonal and hormonal IUDs provide reliable contraception with high rates of efficacy and convenience.

Non-Hormonal IUDs: Non-hormonal IUDs, such as copper-containing devices, prevent pregnancy by creating a hostile environment for sperm, impairing their motility and viability, and inhibiting fertilization. Copper IUDs offer long-term contraception, with typical durations of effectiveness ranging from 5 to 10 years.

Hormonal IUDs: Hormonal IUDs release progestin hormones, such as levonorgestrel, directly into the uterine cavity, exerting contraceptive effects by thickening cervical mucus, inhibiting sperm motility, and thinning the endometrial lining. Hormonal IUDs offer highly effective contraception with typical durations of effectiveness ranging from 3 to 7 years.

Treatment of Gynecological Disorders: In addition to contraception, intrauterine drug delivery systems are utilized in the treatment of various gynecological disorders, providing targeted delivery of therapeutic agents to the uterus and surrounding tissues.

Menorrhagia: Hormonal IUDs, particularly those containing levonorgestrel, are effective in reducing menstrual bleeding and alleviating symptoms of menorrhagia, a common gynecological condition characterized by abnormally heavy or prolonged menstrual bleeding.

Endometriosis: Hormonal IUDs may also be used in the management of endometriosis, a chronic condition characterized by the presence of endometrial tissue outside the uterus. By suppressing endometrial growth and reducing menstrual bleeding, hormonal IUDs can help alleviate pain and other symptoms associated with endometriosis.

Management of Reproductive Health Conditions: Intrauterine drug delivery systems are also employed in the management of various reproductive health conditions, including the prevention of endometrial diseases and the treatment of other uterine disorders.

Endometrial Hyperplasia: Hormonal IUDs, by thinning the endometrial lining and reducing menstrual bleeding, may help prevent endometrial hyperplasia, a condition characterized by abnormal proliferation of endometrial cells and increased risk of endometrial cancer.

Uterine Fibroids: While not a primary treatment modality, hormonal IUDs may provide symptomatic relief for women with uterine fibroids, non-cancerous growths in the uterus that can cause heavy menstrual bleeding and pelvic pain. By reducing menstrual bleeding and suppressing endometrial growth, hormonal IUDs can help manage symptoms associated with uterine fibroids.

This highlights the diverse clinical applications and therapeutic uses of intrauterine drug delivery systems, including contraception, treatment of gynecological disorders, and management of reproductive health conditions. By providing targeted drug delivery to the uterus, IUDs offer effective and convenient solutions for improving women's health outcomes and quality of life.

Challenges and Future Perspectives

Intrauterine drug delivery systems (IUDs) hold immense promise for revolutionizing women's healthcare by offering targeted and long-lasting therapeutic interventions. However, several challenges must be addressed to fully realize their potential and enhance their clinical utility. Additionally, ongoing advancements in technology and evolving patient preferences are shaping the future landscape of IUDs.

Biocompatibility Issues: Ensuring the biocompatibility of intrauterine drug delivery systems is essential to minimize adverse reactions and maximize patient safety. Biocompatibility issues may arise from interactions between the device and the uterine environment, leading to inflammation, infection, or tissue damage. To address these challenges, careful selection of materials and coatings, rigorous preclinical testing, and close monitoring of patient outcomes are necessary. Future developments in biomaterials science and biocompatibility testing methodologies may further enhance the safety and efficacy of IUDs. Reference: Ratner BD, Hoffman AS, Schoen FJ, Lemons JE. Biomaterials science: an introduction to materials in medicine. 3rd ed. London, UK: Elsevier Academic Press; 2013.

Patient Acceptance and Compliance: Despite their effectiveness and convenience, intrauterine drug delivery systems face challenges related to patient acceptance and compliance. Misconceptions, cultural beliefs, and lack of awareness about IUDs may contribute to reluctance among some women to consider them as a contraceptive or therapeutic option. Moreover, concerns about pain during insertion, device expulsion, and side effects may impact patient satisfaction and adherence. To address these issues, education, counseling, and improved access to healthcare services are essential. Additionally, innovations in device design, insertion techniques, and pain management strategies may enhance patient acceptance and compliance with IUDs.

Emerging Trends and Technologies: The field of intrauterine drug delivery systems is witnessing rapid advancements driven by emerging trends and technologies. Novel drug-eluting polymers, biodegradable materials, and microfabrication techniques are expanding the possibilities for designing next-generation IUDs with improved drug release kinetics, biocompatibility, and patient convenience. Additionally, digital health technologies, such as smartphone apps and wearable devices, are being integrated with IUDs to enhance user experience, facilitate remote monitoring, and promote adherence. Furthermore, the development of personalized medicine approaches and targeted drug delivery strategies holds promise for tailoring IUDs to individual patient needs, optimizing therapeutic outcomes, and minimizing side effects.

This note highlights the challenges and future perspectives of intrauterine drug delivery systems, including biocompatibility issues, patient acceptance and compliance, and emerging trends and technologies. By addressing these challenges and leveraging innovative approaches, IUDs have the potential to revolutionize women's healthcare and improve health outcomes on a global scale.

Regulatory Considerations and Market Landscape

Regulatory considerations and market dynamics play pivotal roles in shaping the development, approval, and commercialization of intrauterine drug delivery systems. Understanding the regulatory pathway, market trends, and competitive landscape is crucial for navigating the complex landscape of women's healthcare products.

FDA Approval Process: The Food and Drug Administration (FDA) oversees the regulatory approval process for intrauterine drug delivery systems in the United States. Manufacturers seeking FDA approval must demonstrate the safety, efficacy, and quality of their products through preclinical and clinical studies in accordance with regulatory guidelines.

Preclinical Studies: Preclinical studies involve in vitro and in vivo evaluations of the device's biocompatibility, drug release kinetics, and pharmacokinetic properties. These studies provide essential data to support the rationale for clinical testing and guide formulation optimization.

Clinical Trials: Clinical trials are conducted in phases to assess the safety and efficacy of the intrauterine drug delivery system in human subjects. Phase I trials evaluate safety and tolerability, Phase II trials assess preliminary efficacy and dose-ranging, and Phase III trials confirm efficacy and monitor adverse events in larger patient populations.

FDA Submission: Following successful completion of clinical trials, manufacturers submit a New Drug Application (NDA) or a Biologics License Application (BLA) to the FDA for review. The FDA evaluates the data to determine whether the device meets regulatory standards for safety, efficacy, and quality.

Market Analysis and Trends: The market for intrauterine drug delivery systems is characterized by steady growth driven by increasing demand for long-acting, reversible contraceptive options and innovative therapeutic solutions for gynecological disorders. Key market trends and drivers include:

Growing Demand for Long-Acting Contraception: Rising awareness of the benefits of long-acting reversible contraception (LARC) and efforts to reduce unintended pregnancies are driving demand for intrauterine drug delivery systems as preferred contraceptive options.

Expanding Applications in Gynecological Care: In addition to contraception, intrauterine drug delivery systems are increasingly used in the treatment of gynecological disorders such as menorrhagia, endometriosis, and uterine fibroids, expanding their market potential.

Technological Advancements: Ongoing advancements in materials science, drug delivery technologies, and digital health solutions are driving innovation in the field of intrauterine drug delivery systems, opening up new opportunities for product differentiation and market growth.

Competitive Landscape: The market for intrauterine drug delivery systems is characterized by intense competition among pharmaceutical companies, medical device manufacturers, and healthcare providers. Key players in the market include:

Bayer AG: Bayer AG is a leading manufacturer of hormonal intrauterine drug delivery systems, with products such as Mirena® and Kyleena®. These devices are widely used for contraception and the management of gynecological disorders.

Teva Pharmaceutical Industries Ltd.: Teva Pharmaceutical Industries Ltd. is a prominent supplier of generic intrauterine drug delivery systems, offering cost-effective alternatives to branded products.

Medicines360: Medicines360 is a non-profit pharmaceutical company that develops and distributes affordable intrauterine drug delivery systems, with a focus on expanding access to women's healthcare products in underserved communities.

CooperSurgical, Inc.: CooperSurgical, Inc. specializes in the development and distribution of medical devices for women's healthcare, including a range of intrauterine drug delivery systems for contraception and gynecological care.

This discussion provides insight into the regulatory considerations and market landscape of intrauterine drug delivery systems, covering the FDA approval process, market analysis and trends, and the competitive landscape. By understanding these dynamics, stakeholders can navigate the complexities of product development, regulatory compliance, and market positioning to achieve success in the rapidly evolving field of women's healthcare.

Case Studies and Clinical Trials

Case studies and clinical trials play crucial roles in evaluating the efficacy, safety, and long-term outcomes of intrauterine drug delivery systems. These studies provide valuable insights into the real-world performance of IUDs and inform clinical decision-making.

Efficacy Studies: Efficacy studies assess the contraceptive effectiveness and therapeutic benefits of intrauterine drug delivery systems in diverse patient populations. These studies typically involve controlled clinical trials with predefined endpoints, including pregnancy rates, symptom relief, or disease progression.Case Study: A randomized controlled trial comparing the contraceptive efficacy of a levonorgestrel-releasing intrauterine system (LNG-IUS) versus a copper intrauterine device (Cu-IUD) in women seeking long-term contraception. The study demonstrates that LNG-IUSs provide superior contraceptive effectiveness compared to Cu-IUDs, with lower pregnancy rates and higher user satisfaction over a 5-year follow-up period.

Safety Assessments: Safety assessments evaluate the incidence and severity of adverse events associated with intrauterine drug delivery systems, including device-related complications, side effects, and adverse reactions. These assessments are essential for identifying potential risks and ensuring patient safety.Case Study: A post-marketing surveillance study examining the safety profile of a levonorgestrel-releasing intrauterine system (LNG-IUS) in a large cohort of women using the device for contraception or management of gynecological conditions. The study demonstrates that LNG-IUSs are well-tolerated with low rates of serious adverse events, including perforation, expulsion, and pelvic infection, during long-term use.

Long-term Follow-up: Long-term follow-up studies provide insights into the durability, efficacy, and safety of intrauterine drug delivery systems over extended periods of use. These studies are essential for assessing the persistence of contraceptive effectiveness, symptom relief, or disease control over time.

Case Study: A prospective cohort study evaluating the long-term outcomes of women using a levonorgestrel-releasing intrauterine system (LNG-IUS) for contraception or management of heavy menstrual bleeding.

The study demonstrates sustained contraceptive effectiveness and symptom improvement over a 10-year follow-up period, with low rates of device-related complications and high patient satisfaction

These case studies and considerations illustrate the importance of clinical trials, efficacy studies, safety assessments, and long-term follow-up in evaluating the performance and outcomes of intrauterine drug delivery systems. By generating robust evidence, these studies contribute to informed decision-making, regulatory approval, and clinical practice guidelines, ultimately improving patient care and outcomes in women's health.

Conclusion and Summary

Intrauterine drug delivery systems (IUDs) represent innovative solutions for addressing a wide range of women's healthcare needs, including contraception, treatment of gynecological disorders, and management of reproductive health conditions. Through targeted drug delivery to the uterus, IUDs offer advantages such as long-acting efficacy, convenience, and localized therapeutic effects.

Key Findings and Takeaways

IUDs provide highly effective contraception, with both hormonal and non-hormonal options available to suit individual patient preferences and needs.

In addition to contraception, IUDs offer therapeutic benefits for managing gynecological disorders such as menorrhagia, endometriosis, and uterine fibroids, providing symptom relief and improving quality of life.

Safety assessments and long-term follow-up studies demonstrate that IUDs are generally well-tolerated, with low rates of serious adverse events and high patient satisfaction.

Regulatory considerations, including the FDA approval process, play a critical role in ensuring the safety, efficacy, and quality of IUDs for clinical use.

Market analysis reveals growing demand for IUDs driven by increasing awareness of long-acting contraceptive options and expanding applications in women's healthcare.

Future Directions and Research Opportunities

Further research is needed to optimize the design, formulation, and delivery mechanisms of IUDs to enhance efficacy, safety, and patient acceptance.

Long-term studies are warranted to assess the durability and persistence of contraceptive effectiveness, symptom relief, and disease control with IUDs over extended periods of use.

Emerging technologies, such as drug-eluting polymers, biodegradable materials, and digital health solutions, present opportunities for innovation in the field of intrauterine drug delivery.

Continued collaboration between researchers, clinicians, regulatory agencies, and industry stakeholders is essential for advancing the development and adoption of IUDs in clinical practice.

In summary, intrauterine drug delivery systems offer promising avenues for improving women's health outcomes through targeted and long-lasting therapeutic interventions. By addressing key challenges, leveraging emerging technologies, and fostering interdisciplinary collaboration, the future of IUDs holds great potential for revolutionizing women's healthcare and enhancing quality of life worldwide.

References

Bahamondes L, Hidalgo MM, Bahamondes MV. Intrauterine devices: types, indications, and scientific evidence. Best Pract Res Clin Obstet Gynaecol. 2014;28(8):1113-1123.

Banker GS, Rhodes CT. Modern pharmaceutics. 4th ed. New York, NY: Marcel Dekker; 2002.

Chien YW. Novel drug delivery systems. 2nd ed. New York, NY: Marcel Dekker; 1992.

Frost & Sullivan. Strategic analysis of the global intrauterine contraceptive devices (IUCD) market. Available from: https://store.frost.com/strategic-analysis-of-the-global-intrauterine-contraceptive-devices-iucd-market.html.

Gemzell-Danielsson K, Mansour D, Fiala C, Kaunitz AM, Bahamondes L. Management of pain associated with the insertion of intrauterine contraceptives. Hum Reprod Update. 2013;19(5):419-427.

Gemzell-Danielsson K, Mansour D, Fiala C, Kaunitz AM, Bahamondes L. Management of pain associated with the insertion of intrauterine contraceptives. Hum Reprod Update. 2013;19(5):419-427.

Gemzell-Danielsson K, Mansour D, Fiala C, Kaunitz AM, Bahamondes L. Management of pain associated with the insertion of intrauterine contraceptives. Hum Reprod Update. 2013;19(5):419-427.

Gemzell-Danielsson K, Schellschmidt I, Apter D. A randomized, phase II study describing the efficacy, bleeding profile, and safety of two low-dose levonorgestrel-releasing intrauterine contraceptive systems and Mirena. Fertil Steril. 2012;97(3):616-622.

Gemzell-Danielsson K, Schellschmidt I, Apter D. A randomized, phase II study describing the efficacy, bleeding profile, and safety of two low-dose levonorgestrel-releasing intrauterine contraceptive systems and Mirena. Fertil Steril. 2012;97(3):616-622.

Grand View Research. Intrauterine devices (IUDs) market size, share & trends analysis report by product (copper IUD, hormonal IUD), by end-use (hospitals, clinics), by region (North America, Europe, APAC), and segment forecasts, 2020-2027. Available from: https://www.grandviewresearch.com/industry-analysis/intrauterine-devices-iuds-market.

Guyton AC, Hall JE. Textbook of medical physiology. 13th ed. Philadelphia, PA: Elsevier; 2016.*

Heinemann K, Reed S, Moehner S, Minh TD. Comparative contraceptive effectiveness of levonorgestrel-releasing and copper intrauterine devices: the European Active Surveillance Study for Intrauterine Devices. Contraception. 2015;91(4):280-283.

Lee JK, Parisi SM, Akers AY, et al. The impact of contraceptive counseling in primary care on contraceptive use. J Gen Intern Med. 2011;26(7):731-736.

Maruo T, Ohara N, Yoshida S, et al. Effects of levonorgestrel-releasing intrauterine system on proliferation and apoptosis of cultured human uterine leiomyoma cells. Hum Reprod. 2006;21(2):1-8.

McCoy C, Edward J. Clinical pharmacology: a pharmaceutical professional's guide. 2nd ed. Burlington, MA: Jones & Bartlett Learning; 2018.

McCoy C, Edward J. Clinical pharmacology: a pharmaceutical professional's guide. 2nd ed. Burlington, MA: Jones & Bartlett Learning; 2018.

Modi MN, Gilchrist BF, Shores JH. Levonorgestrel intrauterine system: a pragmatic guide for Mirena. J Am Board Fam Pract. 2003;16(2):161-167.

Moore KL, Persaud TVN, Torchia MG. The developing human: clinically oriented embryology. 10th ed. Philadelphia, PA: Saunders; 2016.

Rathbone MJ, Hadgraft J, Roberts MS, Lane ME. Modified-release drug delivery technology. 2nd ed. New York, NY: Informa Healthcare; 2008.

Rathbone MJ, Hadgraft J, Roberts MS, Lane ME. Modified-release drug delivery technology. 2nd ed. New York, NY: Informa Healthcare; 2008.

Ratner BD, Hoffman AS, Schoen FJ, Lemons JE. Biomaterials science: an introduction to materials in medicine. 3rd ed. London, UK: Elsevier Academic Press; 2013.

Reference: Frost & Sullivan. Strategic analysis of the global intrauterine contraceptive devices (IUCD) market. Available from: https://store.frost.com/strategic-analysis-of-the-global-intrauterine-contraceptive-devices-iucd-market.html.

Reference: Grand View Research. Intrauterine devices (IUDs) market size, share & trends analysis report by product (copper IUD, hormonal IUD), by end-use (hospitals, clinics), by region (North America, Europe, APAC), and segment forecasts, 2020-2027. Available from: https://www.grandviewresearch.com/industry-analysis/intrauterine-devices-iuds-market.

Reference: Heinemann K, Reed S, Moehner S, Minh TD. Comparative contraceptive effectiveness of levonorgestrel-releasing and copper intrauterine devices: the European Active Surveillance Study for Intrauterine Devices. Contraception. 2015;91(4):280-283.

Reference: Sivin I, Stern J. Health during prolonged use of levonorgestrel 20 micrograms/d and the copper TCu 380Ag intrauterine contraceptive devices: a multicenter study. International Committee for Contraception Research (ICCR). Contraception. 1991;44(5):473-490.

Reference: U.S. Food and Drug Administration. Guidance for industry: intrauterine contraception: developing an intrauterine contraceptive. Available from: https://www.fda.gov/regulatory-information/search-fda-guidance-documents/intrauterine-contraception-developing-intrauterine-contraceptive.

Rowland M, Tozer TN. Clinical pharmacokinetics and pharmacodynamics: concepts and applications. 5th ed. Philadelphia, PA: Wolters Kluwer Health; 2019.

Rowland M, Tozer TN. Clinical pharmacokinetics and pharmacodynamics: concepts and applications. 5th ed. Philadelphia, PA: Wolters Kluwer Health; 2019.

Siepmann J, Siegel RA, Rathbone MJ. Fundamentals and applications of controlled release drug delivery. 2nd ed. New York, NY: Springer; 2012.

Sivin I, Stern J. Health during prolonged use of levonorgestrel 20 micrograms/d and the copper TCu 380Ag intrauterine contraceptive devices: a multicenter study. International Committee for Contraception Research (ICCR). Contraception. 1991;44(5):473-490.

U.S. Food and Drug Administration. Guidance for industry: intrauterine contraception: developing an intrauterine contraceptive. Available from: https://www.fda.gov/regulatory-information/search-fda-guidance-documents/intrauterine-contraception-developing-intrauterine-contraceptive.

Vercellini P, Frontino G, De Giorgi O, Pietropaolo G, Pasin R, Crosignani PG. Continuous use of an oral contraceptive for endometriosis-associated recurrent dysmenorrhea that does not respond to a cyclic pill regimen. Fertil Steril. 2003;80(3):560-563.

Winner B, Peipert JF, Zhao Q, et al. Effectiveness of long-acting reversible contraception. N Engl J Med. 2012;366(21):1998-2007.

Winner B, Peipert JF, Zhao Q, et al. Effectiveness of long-acting reversible contraception. N Engl J Med. 2012;366(21):1998-2007.

Chapter 12
Principles of Drug Delivery

Drug delivery is a complex process that involves the administration of therapeutic agents to achieve desired pharmacological effects. Understanding the principles of drug delivery is essential for optimizing drug efficacy, safety, and patient outcomes.

Drug Absorption, Distribution, Metabolism, and Excretion (ADME)

The pharmacokinetics of a drug govern its absorption, distribution, metabolism, and excretion within the body, collectively known as ADME.

Absorption: Absorption refers to the process by which a drug enters the bloodstream from its site of administration. The route of administration significantly influences drug absorption, with oral, parenteral, transdermal, and inhalation routes offering distinct absorption kinetics. Factors such as drug solubility, formulation, and physicochemical properties affect the rate and extent of absorption.

Distribution: Following absorption, drugs distribute throughout the body via the bloodstream, reaching target tissues and organs. Distribution is influenced by factors such as drug protein binding, tissue perfusion, and blood-brain barrier permeability. Variability in distribution may lead to differences in drug concentrations at different sites within the body, impacting pharmacological effects.

Metabolism: Metabolic processes occur primarily in the liver, where drugs undergo biotransformation into metabolites that are more easily eliminated from the body. Drug metabolism may involve phase I reactions (e.g., oxidation, reduction, hydrolysis) and phase II reactions (e.g., conjugation), leading to the formation of inactive or active metabolites. Genetic polymorphisms and drug-drug interactions can affect drug metabolism, influencing therapeutic efficacy and toxicity.

Excretion: Excretion involves the elimination of drugs and their metabolites from the body, primarily through renal excretion, hepatic metabolism, and biliary excretion. Other routes of excretion include pulmonary exhalation, sweat, and feces. Renal clearance, hepatic clearance, and half-life are important pharmacokinetic parameters that determine the rate of drug elimination from the body.

Pharmacokinetics and Pharmacodynamics: Pharmacokinetics and pharmacodynamics are fundamental concepts in drug delivery that govern the time course of drug action and the relationship between drug concentration and pharmacological response.

Pharmacokinetics: Pharmacokinetics describes the quantitative analysis of drug absorption, distribution, metabolism, and excretion over time. Pharmacokinetic parameters, such as bioavailability, volume of distribution, clearance, and half-life, characterize the drug's behavior in the body and influence dosing regimens and therapeutic outcomes.

Pharmacodynamics: Pharmacodynamics refers to the study of the biochemical and physiological effects of drugs and their mechanisms of action. Pharmacodynamic parameters, such as potency, efficacy, onset of action, duration of action, and dose-response relationships, determine the therapeutic and adverse effects of drugs on target tissues and cells.

Drug Release Mechanisms: Drug release mechanisms govern the rate and extent of drug release from pharmaceutical dosage forms, influencing the onset, duration, and intensity of pharmacological effects.

Dissolution: Dissolution is the process by which a drug dissolves from its dosage form and becomes available for absorption. Drug dissolution depends on factors such as drug solubility, particle size, and formulation characteristics. Dissolution testing is commonly used to assess the in vitro release of drugs from dosage forms and ensure consistency in drug performance.

Diffusion: Diffusion involves the movement of drug molecules from regions of higher concentration to regions of lower concentration, driven by concentration gradients. Diffusion-based drug release occurs primarily in matrix-type dosage forms, where the drug is dispersed within a polymeric matrix and diffuses out as the matrix erodes or swells.

Dissolution-Controlled Release: In dissolution-controlled release, drug release is governed by the rate of dissolution of the dosage form. Factors such as drug solubility, dosage form design, and dissolution media influence the release rate and profile. Controlled-release formulations, such as extended-release tablets and capsules, aim to maintain therapeutic drug levels over an extended period, reducing dosing frequency and improving patient compliance.

Diffusion-Controlled Release: In diffusion-controlled release, drug release is governed by the rate of diffusion of the drug molecules through a barrier or membrane. Diffusion-based systems, such as transdermal patches and osmotic pumps, control drug release by modulating the permeability of the membrane or the concentration gradient across the membrane.

Understanding the principles of drug delivery is essential for developing safe, effective, and patient-friendly drug delivery systems. By elucidating the mechanisms of drug absorption, distribution, metabolism, and excretion, as well as the kinetics and dynamics of drug action, researchers and clinicians can optimize drug formulations, dosing regimens, and treatment strategies to improve therapeutic outcomes and patient care.

Absorption is a fundamental process in pharmacokinetics that determines the rate and extent to which a drug enters the systemic circulation after administration. Understanding the mechanisms of drug absorption is essential for optimizing drug delivery and achieving therapeutic efficacy.

Introduction to Absorption

Definition and Overview: Absorption refers to the movement of drug molecules from the site of administration into the bloodstream. It is a crucial step in the pharmacokinetic profile of a drug, influencing its bioavailability, onset of action, and therapeutic effects.

Importance of Absorption: Efficient absorption ensures that an adequate concentration of the drug reaches its target site of action, leading to the desired pharmacological response. Factors such as drug solubility, formulation, and route of administration influence the absorption process.

Factors Influencing Drug Absorption

Physicochemical Properties of the Drug: Drug molecules with high lipid solubility and low molecular weight tend to have better absorption rates. Factors such as ionization state, pKa, and partition coefficient impact drug absorption across biological membranes.

Route of Administration: The route of administration significantly affects drug absorption kinetics. Oral, parenteral, transdermal, inhalation, and other routes offer distinct advantages and limitations in terms of absorption efficiency and onset of action.

Formulation Factors: Dosage form design, excipients, and formulation aids influence drug solubility, dissolution, and permeability, thereby affecting absorption. Formulation optimization is critical for enhancing drug bioavailability and therapeutic efficacy.

Physiological Factors: Physiological variables such as gastrointestinal pH, gastrointestinal motility, blood flow, surface area, and membrane permeability influence drug absorption. Variability in these factors may lead to differences in absorption rates among individuals.

Routes of Drug Absorption

Oral Drug Absorption: Oral administration is the most common route of drug delivery, offering convenience and patient compliance. Drug absorption following oral administration occurs primarily in the gastrointestinal tract, where drugs traverse the epithelial barrier of the intestines and enter the systemic circulation.

Parenteral Drug Absorption: Parenteral routes, including intravenous, intramuscular, subcutaneous, and intradermal administration, bypass the gastrointestinal tract and deliver drugs directly into the bloodstream. Parenteral drug absorption is rapid and predictable, making it suitable for drugs with poor oral bioavailability or those requiring immediate therapeutic effects.

Transdermal Drug Absorption: Transdermal drug delivery involves the application of drugs to the skin for systemic absorption. Drugs penetrate the stratum corneum, the outermost layer of the skin, and enter the systemic circulation through passive diffusion or facilitated transport. Transdermal patches offer sustained drug release and steady plasma concentrations over an extended period.

Pulmonary Drug Absorption: Inhalation drug delivery delivers drugs to the lungs for rapid absorption into the bloodstream. Pulmonary drug absorption is efficient due to the large surface area and extensive vascularization of the lungs. Inhalation therapy is commonly used for the treatment of respiratory diseases such as asthma and chronic obstructive pulmonary disease (COPD).

Factors Affecting Oral Drug Absorption

Gastrointestinal Physiology: The gastrointestinal environment, including pH, transit time, and presence of enzymes and transporters, influences drug absorption. Gastric emptying rate and intestinal motility affect the residence time of drugs in the gastrointestinal tract, impacting absorption kinetics.

First-Pass Metabolism: Drugs absorbed from the gastrointestinal tract undergo first-pass metabolism in the liver before entering the systemic circulation. First-pass metabolism may result in significant drug degradation and reduced bioavailability, necessitating higher doses or alternative routes of administration.

Enhancing Drug Absorption

Prodrug Strategies: Prodrugs are inactive or less active drug derivatives that undergo metabolic activation to the active drug moiety following administration. Prodrug formulations improve drug absorption, bioavailability, and therapeutic efficacy by circumventing barriers to absorption and enhancing membrane permeability.

Absorption Enhancers: Absorption enhancers, such as surfactants, bile salts, and penetration enhancers, improve drug absorption by altering membrane permeability and promoting paracellular or transcellular transport. Absorption enhancers are used to overcome biological barriers and enhance drug delivery to target tissues.

Conclusion

Drug absorption is a complex process influenced by various physiological, formulation, and route-dependent factors. Understanding the mechanisms of drug absorption is essential for optimizing drug delivery, enhancing therapeutic efficacy, and improving patient outcomes. Future research in absorption science aims to develop innovative drug delivery strategies, overcome biological barriers, and enhance drug bioavailability for the treatment of various diseases.

Distribution

Distribution is a crucial pharmacokinetic process that determines how drugs are transported throughout the body, from the bloodstream to various tissues and organs. Understanding the mechanisms of drug distribution is essential for optimizing therapy and achieving desired therapeutic outcomes.

Introduction to Distribution

Definition and Overview: Distribution refers to the process by which drugs are transported from the bloodstream to various tissues and organs in the body. It involves the movement of drugs across biological barriers, including cell membranes and tissue compartments, and their distribution in different body compartments.

Importance of Distribution: Distribution plays a critical role in determining the concentration of drugs at their target sites of action, influencing the onset, duration, and intensity of pharmacological effects. Factors such as drug protein binding, tissue perfusion, and blood-brain barrier permeability affect drug distribution kinetics.

Factors Influencing Drug Distribution

Physicochemical Properties of the Drug: Drug properties such as molecular weight, lipid solubility, protein binding affinity, and ionization state influence drug distribution. Lipophilic drugs tend to distribute more readily into tissues, whereas hydrophilic drugs may be restricted to the bloodstream.

Protein Binding: Many drugs bind reversibly to plasma proteins such as albumin and alpha-1 acid glycoprotein, which serve as carriers in the bloodstream. Only the unbound (free) fraction of the drug is pharmacologically active and capable of distributing into tissues. Changes in protein binding can affect the distribution and pharmacological effects of drugs.

Tissue Perfusion: Blood flow to various tissues and organs determines the rate and extent of drug distribution. Highly perfused tissues such as the liver, kidneys, heart, and brain receive a greater supply of blood and thus have higher concentrations of drugs compared to less perfused tissues.

Biological Barriers: Biological barriers such as the blood-brain barrier, placental barrier, and blood-tissue barriers regulate the passage of drugs between the bloodstream and target tissues. Barrier permeability influences drug distribution to specific anatomical sites and compartments.

Distribution Kinetics

Volume of Distribution (Vd): The volume of distribution is a pharmacokinetic parameter that quantifies the apparent volume into which a drug distributes in the body. It represents the theoretical volume required to account for the total amount of drug in the body at a given concentration. Drugs with high Vd values distribute extensively into tissues, whereas drugs with low Vd values remain primarily in the bloodstream.

Tissue Distribution Profiles: Drugs exhibit different tissue distribution profiles based on their physicochemical properties, protein binding characteristics, and tissue perfusion rates. Tissue distribution studies provide insights into the distribution patterns and accumulation of drugs in various organs and tissues over time.

Factors Affecting Drug Distribution

Physiological Variability: Interindividual variability in physiological factors such as tissue perfusion, protein binding capacity, and barrier permeability can affect drug distribution among individuals. Factors such as age, gender, disease states, and genetic polymorphisms may influence drug distribution kinetics and tissue concentrations.

Principles of Drug Delivery

Drug Interactions: Drug-drug interactions can alter the distribution of drugs by affecting protein binding, metabolic pathways, or transporter systems. Concurrent administration of drugs with high protein binding affinity may displace other drugs from plasma proteins, leading to increased free drug concentrations and potential toxicity.

Disease States: Alterations in physiological conditions associated with disease states can impact drug distribution. For example, changes in tissue perfusion, protein binding, or barrier integrity in diseased tissues may affect drug distribution kinetics and therapeutic outcomes.

Clinical Implications of Drug Distribution

Therapeutic Monitoring: Understanding the distribution kinetics of drugs is essential for therapeutic monitoring and dose optimization. Therapeutic drug monitoring involves measuring drug concentrations in blood or tissues to ensure therapeutic efficacy while minimizing toxicity.

Targeted Drug Delivery: Targeted drug delivery strategies aim to enhance drug distribution to specific tissues or organs while minimizing systemic exposure. Nanoparticulate drug carriers, liposomes, and monoclonal antibodies can be engineered to target diseased tissues or cellular receptors, improving drug localization and therapeutic outcomes.

Conclusion

Drug distribution is a dynamic process influenced by various physiological, pharmacological, and patient-specific factors. Understanding the mechanisms of drug distribution is essential for optimizing therapy, achieving desired therapeutic outcomes, and minimizing adverse effects. Future research in drug distribution aims to develop targeted drug delivery systems, overcome biological barriers, and enhance drug localization for the treatment of various diseases.

Metabolism

Metabolism is a crucial pharmacokinetic process that involves the biotransformation of drugs into metabolites, which can be either active or inactive. Understanding drug metabolism is essential for predicting drug interactions, determining dosing regimens, and assessing drug safety and efficacy.

Introduction to Drug Metabolism

Definition and Overview: Drug metabolism refers to the enzymatic conversion of drugs into metabolites, primarily in the liver and other tissues. Metabolism plays a critical role in determining the pharmacokinetics, pharmacodynamics, and therapeutic effects of drugs.

Importance of Drug Metabolism: Metabolism influences the bioavailability, distribution, and elimination of drugs from the body. Metabolites may exhibit different pharmacological activities, toxicity profiles, and elimination kinetics compared to the parent drug.

Phases of Drug Metabolism

Phase I Metabolism: Phase I metabolism involves functionalization reactions such as oxidation, reduction, and hydrolysis, which introduce or unmask functional groups on the drug molecule. Cytochrome P450 enzymes, particularly CYP3A4, CYP2D6, and CYP2C9, play a central role in phase I metabolism.

Phase II Metabolism: Phase II metabolism involves conjugation reactions such as glucuronidation, sulfation, acetylation, and methylation, which conjugate the drug or its phase I metabolites with endogenous molecules to facilitate excretion. Phase II metabolism enhances water solubility and facilitates renal or biliary excretion of metabolites.

Factors Influencing Drug Metabolism

Genetic Factors: Genetic polymorphisms in drug-metabolizing enzymes and drug transporters can lead to interindividual variability in drug metabolism and pharmacokinetics. Poor metabolizer phenotypes may result in reduced drug clearance and increased risk of adverse effects, while ultra-rapid metabolizer phenotypes may lead to subtherapeutic drug levels.

Drug-Drug Interactions: Drug-drug interactions occur when co-administered drugs affect the activity of drug-metabolizing enzymes or transporters, leading to alterations in drug metabolism and pharmacokinetics. Inducers such as rifampicin and inhibitors such as ketoconazole can modulate enzyme activity and influence the metabolism of co-administered drugs.

Physiological Factors: Physiological factors such as age, gender, liver function, renal function, and disease states can influence drug metabolism. Hepatic impairment may reduce the clearance of drugs metabolized by the liver, while renal impairment may affect the excretion of metabolites.

Clinical Implications of Drug Metabolism

Drug Interactions: Understanding drug metabolism is essential for predicting and managing drug interactions. Clinicians should be aware of potential interactions between drugs metabolized by the same enzyme pathways or affected by enzyme inducers or inhibitors.

Pharmacogenomics: Pharmacogenomic testing can identify genetic variants associated with altered drug metabolism and guide personalized drug therapy. Genetic testing may help identify patients at increased risk of adverse drug reactions or therapeutic failure.

Drug Toxicity: Drug metabolism can produce reactive metabolites that may cause drug-induced liver injury or other adverse effects. Knowledge of the metabolic pathways and potential toxic metabolites is critical for drug safety assessment and risk management.

Future Directions in Drug Metabolism

Precision Medicine: Advances in pharmacogenomics and personalized medicine are driving efforts to tailor drug therapy based on individual genetic profiles and metabolic phenotypes. Precision medicine approaches aim to optimize drug selection, dosing, and monitoring to maximize therapeutic efficacy and minimize adverse effects.

Drug Design: Rational drug design strategies consider metabolic stability and clearance pathways during drug development to optimize pharmacokinetic properties and minimize metabolic liabilities. Prodrugs, metabolic inhibitors, and transporter substrates are designed to modulate drug metabolism and enhance therapeutic outcomes.

Drug metabolism is a dynamic and complex process that plays a critical role in drug disposition and pharmacokinetics. Understanding the mechanisms of drug metabolism is essential for optimizing drug therapy, predicting drug interactions, and ensuring patient safety and efficacy. Future research in drug metabolism aims to elucidate novel metabolic pathways, develop predictive models, and advance personalized medicine approaches for improved patient care.

Excretion

Excretion is a vital pharmacokinetic process responsible for the removal of drugs and their metabolites from the body. Understanding the mechanisms of drug excretion is essential for predicting drug clearance, optimizing dosing regimens, and assessing drug safety.

Introduction to Excretion

Definition and Overview: Excretion refers to the elimination of drugs and their metabolites from the body through various routes, including renal excretion, hepatic metabolism, biliary excretion, pulmonary exhalation, and fecal excretion. Excretion is a critical determinant of drug clearance and systemic exposure.

Importance of Excretion: Efficient excretion ensures the elimination of drugs and metabolites from the body, preventing drug accumulation and potential toxicity. Factors such as renal function, hepatic function, and drug properties influence drug excretion kinetics.

Routes of Drug Excretion

Renal Excretion: Renal excretion is the primary route of elimination for many drugs and metabolites. Drugs undergo glomerular filtration, tubular secretion, and tubular reabsorption in the kidneys, with the net result determining renal clearance. Renal excretion is influenced by factors such as glomerular filtration rate, urine pH, and drug-protein binding.

Hepatic Metabolism: Hepatic metabolism is another major route of drug excretion, involving biotransformation reactions that convert drugs into more hydrophilic metabolites suitable for elimination. Metabolites may undergo biliary excretion into the bile ducts, where they are eliminated via feces or reabsorbed into the enterohepatic circulation.

Pulmonary Exhalation: Some volatile or gaseous drugs may be eliminated via pulmonary exhalation through the lungs. Drugs administered via inhalation or volatile anesthetics undergo rapid elimination via the respiratory tract.

Fecal Excretion: Drugs and metabolites may be excreted via feces following biliary excretion into the intestines or direct secretion into the gastrointestinal tract. Fecal excretion is particularly relevant for drugs with poor renal clearance or extensive enterohepatic recirculation.

Factors Influencing Drug Excretion

Renal Function: Renal function plays a critical role in determining the rate and extent of renal excretion. Factors such as glomerular filtration rate, tubular secretion, and tubular reabsorption influence renal clearance and drug excretion kinetics. Renal impairment may impair drug excretion and lead to drug accumulation and toxicity.

Hepatic Function: Hepatic function affects drug metabolism and biliary excretion, which contribute to overall drug clearance. Liver diseases such as cirrhosis and hepatitis may impair hepatic clearance and excretion, leading to altered pharmacokinetics and increased risk of adverse effects.

Urine pH: Urine pH can influence the ionization and renal elimination of drugs. Weak acids are excreted more readily in alkaline urine, whereas weak bases are excreted more readily in acidic urine. Manipulation of urine pH can be used to enhance or reduce the renal excretion of certain drugs.

Drug Properties: Drug properties such as molecular weight, lipid solubility, protein binding, and ionization state influence drug excretion kinetics. Highly lipophilic drugs tend to undergo extensive hepatic metabolism, while hydrophilic drugs are excreted primarily via renal clearance.

Clinical Implications of Drug Excretion

Dosing Adjustments: Knowledge of drug excretion pathways and factors influencing excretion is essential for determining appropriate dosing regimens, particularly in patients with renal or hepatic impairment. Dosing adjustments may be necessary to avoid drug accumulation and minimize the risk of toxicity.

Therapeutic Drug Monitoring: Therapeutic drug monitoring involves measuring drug concentrations in blood or urine to optimize dosing regimens and ensure therapeutic efficacy. Monitoring drug levels allows clinicians to adjust doses based on individual patient factors and optimize drug therapy.

Drug-Drug Interactions: Drug-drug interactions can affect drug excretion by altering renal clearance, hepatic metabolism, or biliary excretion. Concurrent administration of drugs that compete for renal tubular secretion or hepatic metabolism may lead to changes in drug clearance and potential toxicity.

Future Directions in Drug Excretion

Biomarkers of Renal Function: Biomarkers such as serum creatinine, estimated glomerular filtration rate (eGFR), and urinary albumin-to-creatinine ratio (ACR) are used to assess renal function and predict drug excretion in clinical practice. Future research aims to identify novel biomarkers of renal function for improved prediction of drug clearance and dosing optimization.

Precision Medicine: Advances in pharmacogenomics and personalized medicine may lead to individualized dosing regimens based on genetic factors influencing drug metabolism and excretion. Pharmacogenomic testing can identify patients at increased risk of altered drug clearance and guide personalized drug therapy.

Drug excretion is a multifaceted process influenced by renal function, hepatic function, drug properties, and physiological factors. Understanding the mechanisms of drug excretion is essential for optimizing drug therapy, ensuring patient safety, and minimizing the risk of adverse effects. Future research in drug excretion aims to develop predictive models, biomarkers, and personalized medicine approaches for improved drug dosing and patient care.

Pharmacokinetics and Pharmacodynamics

Introduction to Pharmacokinetics and Pharmacodynamics

Pharmacokinetics (PK) and pharmacodynamics (PD) are fundamental concepts in pharmacology that describe the time course of drug action and the relationship between drug concentration and pharmacological response.

PK focuses on the absorption, distribution, metabolism, and excretion (ADME) of drugs within the body, while PD examines the biochemical and physiological effects of drugs on target tissues and cells.

Pharmacokinetics (PK)

Absorption: Absorption refers to the process by which a drug enters the bloodstream from its site of administration. Factors influencing absorption include route of administration, drug solubility, formulation, and physiological variables.

Distribution: Distribution involves the transport of drugs from the bloodstream to various tissues and organs. Distribution is influenced by factors such as tissue perfusion, protein binding, and membrane permeability.

Metabolism: Metabolism refers to the biotransformation of drugs into metabolites, primarily in the liver and other tissues. Drug metabolism involves phase I and phase II reactions, which enhance drug elimination and facilitate excretion.

Excretion: Excretion is the elimination of drugs and metabolites from the body through renal excretion, hepatic metabolism, biliary excretion, pulmonary exhalation, and fecal excretion. Factors affecting excretion include renal function, hepatic function, and drug properties.

Pharmacodynamics (PD)

Dose-Response Relationship: The dose-response relationship describes the relationship between drug dose and pharmacological response. It includes parameters such as potency, efficacy, and maximal response.

Mechanism of Action: The mechanism of action elucidates how drugs interact with target receptors, enzymes, or ion channels to produce pharmacological effects. Agonists, antagonists, and modulators exert their effects through different mechanisms.

Onset and Duration of Action: The onset of action refers to the time taken for a drug to produce a pharmacological effect, while the duration of action describes the duration of the drug's effect. Factors influencing onset and duration of action include drug concentration, receptor binding kinetics, and tissue distribution.

Variability in Response: Interindividual variability in drug response can arise from genetic factors, physiological differences, drug interactions, and disease states. Understanding variability in drug response is essential for individualizing therapy and optimizing patient outcomes.

Pharmacokinetic-Pharmacodynamic (PK-PD) Modeling

PK-PD modeling integrates pharmacokinetic and pharmacodynamic data to characterize the relationship between drug exposure and response. It allows for the prediction of drug effects at different doses and dosing regimens.

PK-PD modeling can be used to optimize drug dosing, predict therapeutic outcomes, and assess the impact of patient factors on drug response. It is particularly useful in drug development and dose selection.

Clinical Applications

Therapeutic Drug Monitoring (TDM): TDM involves measuring drug concentrations in blood or tissues to optimize dosing regimens and ensure therapeutic efficacy. TDM is used for drugs with narrow therapeutic windows, variable pharmacokinetics, or potential for drug interactions.

Individualized Therapy: PK-PD principles are applied to individualize drug therapy based on patient factors such as age, weight, renal function, and genetic polymorphisms. Individualized therapy aims to maximize therapeutic efficacy while minimizing adverse effects.

Drug Development: PK-PD studies are integral to drug development and regulatory approval processes. They provide insights into drug pharmacokinetics, pharmacodynamics, and safety profiles, guiding dose selection, dosing regimens, and patient selection in clinical trials.

Future Directions

Precision Medicine: Advances in pharmacogenomics, biomarkers, and personalized medicine are driving efforts to tailor drug therapy based on individual patient characteristics. Precision medicine aims to optimize drug selection, dosing, and monitoring to maximize therapeutic efficacy and minimize adverse effects.

Systems Pharmacology: Systems pharmacology integrates computational modeling, omics technologies, and network analysis to elucidate complex drug-disease interactions. It provides a holistic understanding of drug action and disease mechanisms, facilitating the development of novel therapeutics and treatment strategies.

Conclusion

PK and PD are integral concepts in pharmacology that govern the time course of drug action and the relationship between drug concentration and pharmacological response. Understanding PK-PD principles is essential for optimizing drug therapy, individualizing treatment, and advancing precision medicine initiatives. Future research aims to enhance our understanding of drug kinetics and dynamics, improve predictive modeling approaches, and translate findings into clinical practice for improved patient care.

Drug Release Mechanisms

Introduction to Drug Release Mechanisms

Drug release mechanisms describe the processes by which drugs are liberated from pharmaceutical dosage forms and become available for absorption in the body. Understanding these mechanisms is crucial for designing drug delivery systems with controlled release profiles tailored to specific therapeutic needs.

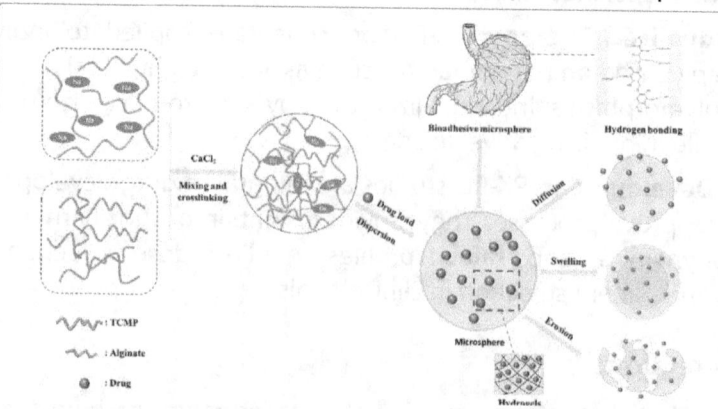

Fig: Drug administration and Drug Release

Dissolution-Controlled Release

In dissolution-controlled release, drug liberation occurs through the dissolution of the dosage form matrix or carrier material. Factors influencing dissolution include drug solubility, particle size, dosage form design, and environmental conditions such as pH and temperature. Rate-controlling polymers or hydrophilic matrices can modulate drug release kinetics by controlling the diffusion of drug molecules out of the dosage form.

Diffusion-Controlled Release

Diffusion-controlled release relies on the diffusion of drug molecules through a barrier or membrane to reach the surrounding medium. The rate of drug diffusion is governed by Fick's laws of diffusion, which describe the movement of molecules from areas of high concentration to low concentration across a concentration gradient. Membrane permeability, thickness, and surface area influence drug diffusion rates and release kinetics.

Osmotic-Controlled Release

Osmotic-controlled release utilizes osmotic pressure gradients to drive drug release from the dosage form. Osmotic pumps or devices contain an osmotically active core surrounded by a semipermeable membrane. Water influx into the core creates pressure, forcing drug solution or suspension out of the delivery orifice at a controlled rate. Osmotic-controlled release systems offer zero-order release kinetics and consistent drug delivery over an extended period.

Ion-Exchange Controlled Release

Ion-exchange controlled release involves the exchange of ions between the drug reservoir and the surrounding medium, leading to controlled drug release. Ion-exchange resins or matrices can be incorporated into the dosage form to facilitate ion exchange and modulate drug release kinetics. Factors such as ion concentration, pH, and ionic strength influence the rate and extent of ion exchange and drug release.

Mechanically-Controlled Release

Mechanically-controlled release mechanisms rely on external stimuli or mechanical forces to trigger drug release from the dosage form. Examples include pH-responsive hydrogels, temperature-sensitive polymers, and stimuli-responsive nanoparticles. External stimuli such as pH changes, temperature variations, light exposure, or mechanical deformation can trigger drug release by inducing changes in the physical or chemical properties of the dosage form.

Combined Release Mechanisms

Many drug delivery systems employ a combination of release mechanisms to achieve desired release profiles. For example, a formulation may utilize both diffusion-controlled and osmotic-controlled release mechanisms to achieve sustained drug delivery with zero-order kinetics. By leveraging multiple release mechanisms, drug delivery systems can optimize drug release profiles to meet specific therapeutic objectives.

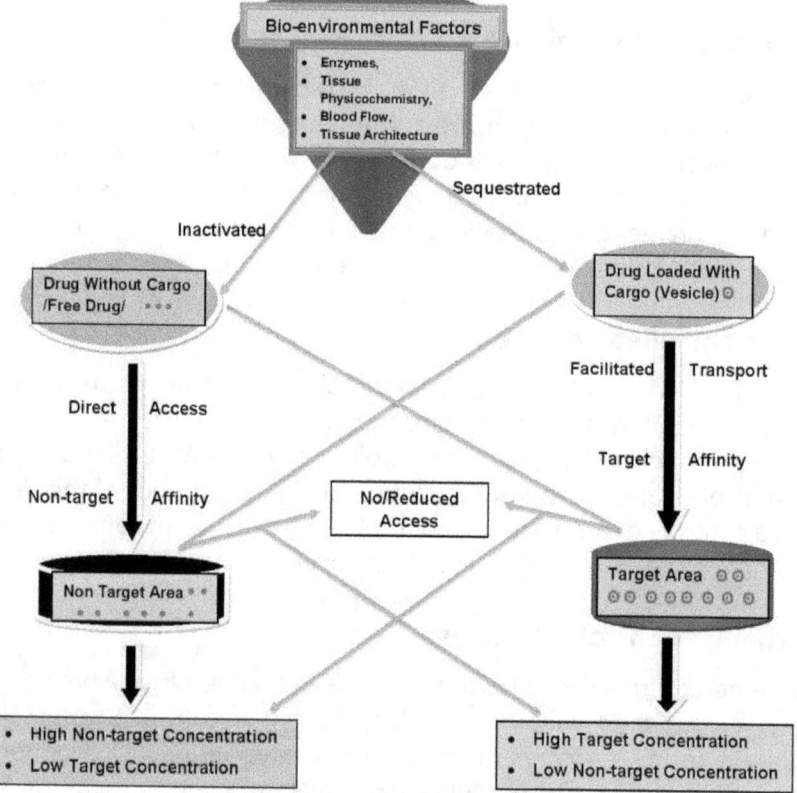

Fig: Drug Targeting

Applications and Clinical Relevance

Drug release mechanisms play a critical role in the design of various drug delivery systems, including oral tablets, capsules, transdermal patches, implants, and injectable depots. Controlled release formulations offer several clinical advantages, including improved patient compliance, reduced dosing frequency, minimized side effects, and enhanced therapeutic efficacy. By tailoring drug release profiles to match physiological needs, controlled release formulations optimize drug therapy and improve patient outcomes.

Challenges and Future Directions

Despite significant progress in drug delivery technology, challenges remain in achieving precise control over drug release kinetics, ensuring formulation stability, and addressing patient variability. Future research aims to develop innovative drug delivery systems with advanced release mechanisms, incorporate novel materials and technologies, and optimize formulation strategies to overcome existing challenges and meet evolving therapeutic needs.

Conclusion

Drug release mechanisms are central to the design and development of controlled release drug delivery systems. By understanding the underlying principles governing drug release, researchers and clinicians can design formulations with tailored release profiles to optimize drug therapy, improve patient outcomes, and address unmet medical needs. Continued advancements in drug delivery technology hold promise for enhancing therapeutic efficacy, minimizing side effects, and improving patient quality of life.

References

Bajpai, S. K., & Sharma, S. (2014). Investigation of pH-sensitive and thermosensitive properties of Poly(N-isopropylacrylamide) and acrylic acid based hydrogels. Smart Materials and Structures, 23(10), 105013.

Brunton, L. L., Hilal-Dandan, R., & Knollmann, B. C. (Eds.). (2018). Goodman & Gilman's: the pharmacological basis of therapeutics. McGraw Hill Professional.

Bruschi, M. L. (2015). Strategies to Modify the Drug Release from Pharmaceutical Systems. Woodhead Publishing.

D'Argenio, D. Z., & Schumitzky, A. (2009). ADME and translational pharmacokinetics/pharmacodynamics of therapeutic proteins: applications in drug discovery and development. Springer Science & Business Media.

D'Argenio, D. Z., & Schumitzky, A. (2009). ADME and translational pharmacokinetics/ pharmacodynamics of therapeutic proteins: applications in drug discovery and development. Springer Science & Business Media.

Evans, W. E., & Schentag, J. J. (1992). Applied pharmacokinetics: principles of therapeutic drug monitoring. Applied Therapeutics.

Gibaldi, M., & Perrier, D. (1982). Pharmacokinetics (Vol. 11). New York: Marcel Dekker.

Hall, J. E. (2015). Guyton and Hall textbook of medical physiology. Elsevier Health Sciences.

Heller, J. (2002). Polymeric controlled release systems: promises, promises. Advanced Drug Delivery Reviews, 54(1), 1-2.

Jansson, B., & Borga, O. (2011). Drug excretion and drug metabolism in the elderly. Gerontology, 27(3), 163-167.

Klaassen, C. D., & Watkins III, J. B. (2015). Casarett & Doull's essentials of toxicology. McGraw Hill Professional.

Langer, R. S., & Peppas, N. A. (1983). Present and future applications of biomaterials in controlled drug delivery systems. Biomaterials, 4(3), 201-214.

Lea, M. A., & Nicholas, P. (1990). Principles of clinical pharmacology. Wiley.

Nies, A. S., & Shand, D. G. (2002). Plumb's Veterinary Drug Handbook: Pocket (5th ed.). Blackwell Science.

Paine, M. F., & Hart, H. L. (2008). Handbook of drug interactions: a clinical and forensic guide. Humana Press.

Peppas, N. A., & Sahlin, J. J. (1996). A simple equation for the description of solute release. II. Fickian and anomalous release from swellable devices. Journal of Controlled Release, 5(37), 123-136.

Rathbone, M. J., Hadgraft, J., & Roberts, M. S. (2008). Modified-Release Drug Delivery Technology. CRC Press.

Ritschel, W. A., Kearns, G. L., & Gibaldi, M. (2013). Handbook of basic pharmacokinetics, including clinical applications. American Pharmaceutical Association.

Ritschel, W. A., Kearns, G. L., & Gibaldi, M. (2013). Handbook of basic pharmacokinetics, including clinical applications. American Pharmaceutical Association.

Robinson, J. R., & Lee, V. H. (2003). Controlled Drug Delivery: Fundamentals and Applications. CRC Press.

Rowland, M., & Tozer, T. N. (2011). Clinical pharmacokinetics and pharmacodynamics: concepts and applications. Lippincott Williams & Wilkins.

Rowland, M., & Tozer, T. N. (2011). Clinical pharmacokinetics and pharmacodynamics: concepts and applications. Lippincott Williams & Wilkins.

Siepmann, J., & Siegel, R. A. (2012). Mathematical modeling of controlled drug delivery. Advanced Drug Delivery Reviews, 64, 83-101.

Smart, J. D. (2005). The basics and underlying mechanisms of mucoadhesion. Advanced Drug Delivery Reviews, 57(11), 1556-1568.

Soppimath, K. S., Aminabhavi, T. M., Kulkarni, A. R., & Rudzinski, W. E. (2001). Biodegradable polymeric nanoparticles as drug delivery devices. Journal of Controlled Release, 70(1-2), 1-20.

Stahl, S. M. (2013). Stahl's essential psychopharmacology: Neuroscientific basis and practical applications. Cambridge University Press.

Tett, S. E., & Kirkpatrick, C. M. (1992). Clinical pharmacokinetics: pocket reference. Anshan.

Wagner, J. G. (1975). Fundamentals of clinical pharmacokinetics. Drug Intelligence Publications.

Zamek-Gliszczynski, M. J., Chu, X., Polli, J. W., Paine, M. F., Galetin, A., & Hsu, V. (2018). Transporters in drug development: discovery, optimization, clinical study and regulation. AAPS journal, 20(3), 1-11.

Zhang, L., & Ma, P. (2017). Understanding drug transport and metabolism: integrating biochemistry and physiology. John Wiley & Sons.

Chapter 13
Emerging Trends and Technologies in Novel Drug Delivery Systems

Introduction to Emerging Trends

Emerging trends and technologies in novel drug delivery systems are shaping the future of pharmaceuticals, offering innovative solutions to improve drug efficacy, safety, and patient compliance. This chapter explores recent advancements and promising developments in drug delivery technology.

Nanotechnology and Nanomedicine

Nanotechnology has revolutionized drug delivery by enabling the design and development of nanoscale drug delivery systems such as nanoparticles, liposomes, and nanofibers. These nanostructures offer advantages such as enhanced drug solubility, targeted delivery, sustained release, and reduced toxicity. Nanomedicine applications include cancer therapy, gene delivery, diagnostic imaging, and regenerative medicine.

Advanced Biomaterials and Polymers

Advances in biomaterials science have led to the development of novel polymers and hydrogels with tailored properties for drug delivery applications. Smart polymers responsive to external stimuli such as pH, temperature, and light offer controlled release capabilities and on-demand drug delivery. Biodegradable and biocompatible polymers enable sustained drug release and tissue regeneration in implantable devices and tissue engineering scaffolds.

Targeted Drug Delivery Systems

Targeted drug delivery systems aim to deliver drugs selectively to diseased tissues or cells while minimizing off-target effects and systemic toxicity. Strategies include ligand-targeted nanoparticles, antibody-drug conjugates, and stimuli-responsive carriers that exploit pathological features such as overexpressed receptors, tumor microenvironment, or intracellular signaling pathways. Targeted delivery enhances drug accumulation at the site of action, improving therapeutic efficacy and reducing side effects.

Personalized Medicine and Pharmacogenomics

Personalized medicine approaches leverage pharmacogenomic information and patient-specific factors to customize drug therapy based on individual genetic profiles, disease characteristics, and treatment responses. Pharmacogenomic testing identifies genetic variants associated with drug metabolism, efficacy, and adverse effects, guiding drug selection, dosing, and monitoring. Personalized drug delivery systems offer tailored dosing regimens and treatment options for improved patient outcomes.

Gene and Cell Therapy Delivery

Gene and cell therapy hold promise for treating genetic disorders, cancer, and regenerative medicine applications. Advanced delivery systems such as viral vectors, lipid nanoparticles, and polymeric carriers enable safe and efficient delivery of therapeutic genes, RNA molecules, or cell-based therapies to target tissues or organs. Gene editing technologies such as CRISPR/Cas9 offer precise genome manipulation for therapeutic intervention in genetic diseases.

Microfluidics and Lab-on-a-Chip Technology

Microfluidic platforms and lab-on-a-chip devices enable precise control and manipulation of fluids at the microscale, facilitating high-throughput screening, drug formulation, and point-of-care diagnostics. Microfluidic systems offer advantages such as reduced sample volumes, rapid analysis, automation, and integration of multiple functions on a single chip. Applications include drug discovery, pharmacokinetic studies, and personalized diagnostics.

Artificial Intelligence and Machine Learning

Artificial intelligence (AI) and machine learning algorithms are transforming drug discovery, formulation design, and clinical decision-making in drug delivery. AI-based approaches analyze large datasets, predict drug properties, optimize formulation parameters, and design customized therapies based on patient data. AI-driven drug delivery systems offer improved drug design, dosage optimization, and real-time monitoring of patient responses.

Regulatory Considerations and Commercialization:

As emerging technologies in drug delivery continue to evolve, regulatory agencies face challenges in evaluating safety, efficacy, and quality standards for novel drug delivery systems. Regulatory considerations include product characterization, stability testing, manufacturing processes, and clinical trial design. Commercialization strategies involve intellectual property protection, market access, reimbursement, and strategic partnerships with industry stakeholders.

Emerging trends and technologies in novel drug delivery systems hold tremendous potential to address unmet medical needs, improve patient outcomes, and advance the field of therapeutics. Future research directions focus on overcoming technical challenges, translating innovations into clinical practice, and harnessing interdisciplinary collaborations to accelerate drug development and healthcare innovation. Continued investment in research, education, and infrastructure is essential to realize the full benefits of emerging drug delivery technologies.

Introduction to Nanotechnology and Nanoparticles

Nanotechnology involves the manipulation of materials at the nanoscale (1-100 nanometers) to create novel structures with unique properties and functionalities. Nanoparticles, one of the most prominent applications of nanotechnology in drug delivery, offer advantages such as high surface area, tunable size and shape, biocompatibility, and the ability to encapsulate drugs for targeted delivery.

Types of Nanoparticles

Liposomes: Liposomes are spherical vesicles composed of lipid bilayers that can encapsulate both hydrophilic and hydrophobic drugs. Liposomal formulations protect drugs from degradation, enhance bioavailability, and enable targeted delivery to specific tissues or cells.

Polymeric Nanoparticles: Polymeric nanoparticles are fabricated from biodegradable or biocompatible polymers such as poly(lactic-co-glycolic acid) (PLGA), polyethylene glycol (PEG), or chitosan. These nanoparticles offer controlled drug release, improved stability, and the potential for site-specific delivery through surface modification or functionalization.

Micelles: Micelles are self-assembled structures formed by amphiphilic molecules in aqueous solution. Micelles can solubilize hydrophobic drugs in their core and improve drug delivery to target tissues. Surface modification with targeting ligands enhances the specificity and efficacy of micellar drug delivery systems.

Nanocrystals: Nanocrystals are crystalline nanoparticles with a size range of 10-1000 nanometers. Nanocrystal formulations improve drug solubility, dissolution rate, and bioavailability, particularly for poorly water-soluble drugs. Nanocrystals exhibit enhanced drug loading capacity and prolonged release kinetics compared to conventional dosage forms.

Dendrimers: Dendrimers are highly branched, symmetric molecules with well-defined structures and multivalent functional groups. Dendrimers can encapsulate drugs, target specific cell types, and facilitate controlled drug release. Surface modification with ligands or antibodies enhances dendrimer-based drug delivery and imaging applications.

Applications of Nanoparticles in Drug Delivery

Cancer Therapy: Nanoparticles play a crucial role in cancer therapy by improving drug delivery to tumor tissues, reducing systemic toxicity, and overcoming multidrug resistance. Targeted nanoparticles deliver chemotherapeutic agents, siRNA, or imaging contrast agents to tumor cells while sparing healthy tissues.

Central Nervous System (CNS) Delivery: Nanoparticles enable drug delivery across the blood-brain barrier (BBB) for the treatment of neurological disorders such as Alzheimer's disease, Parkinson's disease, and brain tumors. Surface modification with BBB-targeting ligands enhances nanoparticle penetration and drug accumulation in the brain.

Vaccine Delivery: Nanoparticles serve as effective carriers for vaccine antigens, adjuvants, and immunomodulatory agents. Nanoparticle-based vaccines enhance antigen stability, promote antigen presentation, and stimulate robust immune responses, offering potential applications in infectious disease prevention and cancer immunotherapy.

Gene Therapy: Nanoparticles facilitate the delivery of nucleic acid therapeutics such as plasmid DNA, mRNA, and small interfering RNA (siRNA) for gene editing, gene silencing, and gene expression modulation. Nanoparticle-mediated gene delivery enhances transfection efficiency, reduces off-target effects, and enables targeted gene delivery to specific cell types or tissues.

Challenges and Considerations

Biocompatibility and Safety: Biocompatibility and safety concerns, including cytotoxicity, immunogenicity, and long-term effects of nanoparticles on biological systems, require thorough evaluation in preclinical and clinical studies.

Scale-up and Manufacturing: Scale-up and manufacturing processes for nanoparticle formulations pose challenges related to reproducibility, batch-to-batch consistency, and regulatory compliance. Optimization of manufacturing techniques and quality control measures are essential for commercial translation.

Regulatory Approval: Regulatory approval pathways for nanoparticle-based drug delivery systems involve addressing complex requirements related to formulation characterization, stability, pharmacokinetics, and toxicity profiles. Collaboration with regulatory agencies is critical for navigating the approval process and ensuring compliance with regulatory standards.

Clinical Translation: Clinical translation of nanoparticle-based drug delivery systems requires rigorous evaluation of safety, efficacy, pharmacokinetics, and pharmacodynamics in human subjects. Clinical trials aim to validate the therapeutic benefits of nanoparticle formulations and establish their clinical utility in diverse disease indications.

Future Perspectives and Outlook

Despite existing challenges, nanotechnology and nanoparticles hold tremendous promise for advancing drug delivery and addressing unmet medical needs. Future research directions focus on harnessing the full potential of nanoparticles for personalized medicine, targeted therapy, and precision drug delivery. Continued interdisciplinary collaboration, innovation, and investment in nanomedicine research are essential for realizing the transformative impact of nanoparticles in healthcare.

Nanotechnology and nanoparticles represent a paradigm shift in drug delivery, offering unprecedented opportunities to improve therapeutic outcomes, enhance patient care, and transform the treatment of diseases. As nanoparticle-based drug delivery systems continue to evolve, they hold the potential to revolutionize the field of medicine and shape the future of healthcare delivery.

Advanced Biomaterials and Polymers in Drug Delivery

Introduction to Advanced Biomaterials and Polymers

Advanced biomaterials and polymers play a pivotal role in drug delivery by providing carriers and matrices for controlled release, targeted delivery, and tissue regeneration. This chapter explores the diverse applications of biomaterials and polymers in drug delivery systems.

Types of Biomaterials and Polymers

Natural Polymers: Natural polymers such as chitosan, alginate, hyaluronic acid, and collagen are derived from biological sources and offer biocompatibility, biodegradability, and low immunogenicity. These polymers are widely used in drug delivery, tissue engineering, and regenerative medicine applications.

Synthetic Polymers: Synthetic polymers such as poly(lactic-co-glycolic acid) (PLGA), polyethylene glycol (PEG), and poly(ε-caprolactone) (PCL) are designed with precise chemical compositions and properties to meet specific requirements in drug delivery systems. Synthetic polymers offer tunable degradation rates, mechanical properties, and drug release kinetics.

Hybrid Biomaterials: Hybrid biomaterials combine natural and synthetic components to leverage the advantages of both materials. Examples include polymer blends, copolymers, and composite materials that exhibit enhanced biocompatibility, mechanical strength, and controlled drug release properties.

Applications of Biomaterials and Polymers in Drug Delivery

Sustained Release Formulations: Biomaterials and polymers enable the development of sustained release formulations that prolong drug release and reduce dosing frequency. Controlled release systems such as microparticles, nanoparticles, and hydrogels provide sustained therapeutic levels of drugs over extended periods, enhancing patient compliance and therapeutic efficacy.

Targeted Drug Delivery Systems: Biomaterial-based targeted drug delivery systems deliver drugs selectively to specific tissues, cells, or organs while minimizing off-target effects and systemic toxicity. Surface modification of biomaterial carriers with targeting ligands, antibodies, or peptides enables precise delivery to diseased sites, improving therapeutic outcomes.

Implantable Devices: Biomaterial implants, such as drug-eluting stents, intraocular implants, and contraceptive devices, provide localized drug delivery for prolonged periods. Biodegradable polymers facilitate the controlled release of drugs from implantable devices, reducing the need for frequent interventions and enhancing patient convenience.

Tissue Engineering Scaffolds: Biomaterial scaffolds support cell growth, proliferation, and tissue regeneration in tissue engineering applications. Porous scaffolds made from biodegradable polymers provide a three-dimensional framework for cell infiltration and extracellular matrix deposition, promoting tissue repair and regeneration in damaged or diseased tissues.

Surface Modification and Functionalization

Surface modification techniques such as chemical conjugation, physical adsorption, and layer-by-layer assembly enable the functionalization of biomaterial surfaces with bioactive molecules, targeting ligands, and stimuli-responsive moieties. Surface-modified biomaterials enhance biocompatibility, cell adhesion, and drug loading capacity, facilitating specific interactions with biological systems.

Challenges and Considerations

Biocompatibility and Cytotoxicity: Biocompatibility assessment and cytotoxicity evaluation are critical considerations in biomaterial design and development. Understanding the interaction of biomaterials with biological systems is essential for ensuring safety and minimizing adverse reactions.

Degradation Kinetics: Biomaterial degradation kinetics influence drug release profiles, tissue response, and long-term biocompatibility. Balancing degradation rates with desired therapeutic outcomes is essential for designing biomaterial-based drug delivery systems with optimal performance.

Regulatory Compliance: Regulatory requirements for biomaterial-based drug delivery systems encompass product characterization, stability testing, manufacturing processes, and preclinical safety assessments. Compliance with regulatory standards ensures product quality, efficacy, and safety for clinical translation.

Future Perspectives and Outlook

Advances in biomaterials science and polymer engineering hold promise for addressing unmet medical needs and advancing drug delivery technology. Future research directions focus on developing multifunctional biomaterials, integrating theranostic capabilities, and translating innovative drug delivery systems from bench to bedside. Continued interdisciplinary collaboration, innovation, and investment in biomaterials research are essential for driving the next generation of drug delivery solutions.

Advanced biomaterials and polymers represent versatile platforms for drug delivery, offering tailored solutions for controlled release, targeted therapy, and tissue regeneration. By harnessing the unique properties of biomaterials and polymers, researchers and clinicians can overcome therapeutic challenges, improve patient outcomes, and advance the field of drug delivery and regenerative medicine.

Personalized Medicine and Pharmacogenomics

Introduction to Personalized Medicine

Personalized medicine, also known as precision medicine, aims to tailor medical treatment to individual characteristics such as genetic makeup, lifestyle, and environmental factors. This chapter explores the principles and applications of personalized medicine, with a focus on pharmacogenomics—the study of how genetic variations influence drug response.

Principles of Pharmacogenomics

Pharmacogenomics investigates how genetic variations in drug metabolism enzymes, drug transporters, and drug targets impact drug efficacy, toxicity, and adverse reactions. Variations in genes encoding cytochrome P450 enzymes (e.g., CYP2D6, CYP2C9) and drug transporters (e.g., ABCB1, SLCO1B1) can affect drug metabolism, absorption, distribution, and excretion, leading to inter-individual differences in drug response.

Genetic Variation and Drug Response

Genetic polymorphisms can alter drug pharmacokinetics (e.g., metabolism, absorption, distribution) and pharmacodynamics (e.g., drug-receptor interactions, downstream signaling pathways). Examples include variations in genes encoding drug-metabolizing enzymes (e.g., poor metabolizers, ultra-rapid metabolizers), drug transporters (e.g., altered substrate specificity), and drug targets (e.g., altered drug binding affinity).

Clinical Applications of Pharmacogenomics

Pharmacogenomic testing enables healthcare providers to predict individual responses to medications, optimize drug selection and dosing, and minimize the risk of adverse drug reactions. Clinical applications include:

Dosing Optimization: Tailoring drug doses based on genetic factors to achieve optimal therapeutic outcomes while minimizing side effects. Examples include warfarin dosing based on CYP2C9 and VKORC1 genotypes, and thiopurine dosing based on TPMT genotype.

Drug Selection: Choosing medications with favorable pharmacogenomic profiles based on individual genetic characteristics. Examples include selecting antidepressants based on CYP2D6 genotype and antiplatelet therapy based on CYP2C19 genotype in patients undergoing percutaneous coronary intervention.

Risk Prediction: Identifying individuals at increased risk of adverse drug reactions or treatment failure based on genetic susceptibility factors. Examples include identifying HLA-B5701 carriers at risk of abacavir hypersensitivity and HLA-B1502 carriers at risk of carbamazepine-induced Stevens-Johnson syndrome.

Challenges and Considerations

Despite the promise of pharmacogenomics in personalized medicine, several challenges remain:

Genetic Complexity: Genetic contributions to drug response are influenced by multiple genes, environmental factors, and gene-environment interactions, making interpretation and prediction complex.

Clinical Implementation: Integrating pharmacogenomic testing into routine clinical practice requires addressing challenges related to test availability, reimbursement, clinician education, and patient acceptance.

Ethical, Legal, and Social Implications: Ethical considerations include privacy, informed consent, and potential discrimination based on genetic information. Legal and regulatory frameworks are needed to ensure responsible use of pharmacogenomic data and protect patient rights.

Future Directions and Opportunities

Advances in genomic technologies, bioinformatics, and data analytics hold promise for overcoming current challenges and expanding the scope of personalized medicine. Future research directions include:

Multi-omics Integration: Integrating genomic, transcriptomic, proteomic, and metabolomic data to provide a comprehensive understanding of drug response mechanisms and identify predictive biomarkers.

Artificial Intelligence and Machine Learning: Leveraging AI and machine learning algorithms to analyze large-scale genomic data, predict drug responses, and optimize treatment strategies in real time.

Patient Engagement and Education: Empowering patients with personalized genomic information, education, and decision support tools to actively participate in treatment decisions and improve health outcomes.

Personalized medicine and pharmacogenomics represent a paradigm shift in healthcare, offering tailored treatment approaches based on individual genetic characteristics. By integrating genomic information into clinical practice, healthcare providers can optimize drug therapy, minimize adverse effects, and improve patient outcomes in the era of precision medicine. Continued research, education, and collaboration are essential for realizing the full potential of personalized medicine in transforming healthcare delivery.

Gene and Cell Therapy Delivery

Introduction to Gene and Cell Therapy

Gene and cell therapy are innovative approaches that involve the delivery of genetic material or cells to modulate cellular functions, correct genetic defects, or regenerate damaged tissues. This chapter explores the principles and applications of gene and cell therapy delivery systems in the treatment of genetic disorders, cancer, and other diseases.

Gene Delivery Systems

Viral Vectors: Viral vectors, derived from viruses such as retroviruses, lentiviruses, adenoviruses, and adeno-associated viruses (AAVs), are commonly used for gene delivery due to their high transduction efficiency and ability to integrate genetic material into host cells. Viral vectors can deliver therapeutic genes to target cells, enabling gene replacement, gene correction, or gene silencing approaches.

Non-viral Vectors: Non-viral vectors, including liposomes, polymers, and nanoparticles, offer advantages such as low immunogenicity, ease of manufacturing, and flexibility in cargo delivery. Non-viral vectors can deliver plasmid DNA, mRNA, or small interfering RNA (siRNA) to target cells, providing transient or sustained gene expression without genomic integration.

Cell Therapy Delivery Systems

Stem Cell Therapy: Stem cell therapy involves the transplantation of stem cells or progenitor cells into damaged tissues to promote tissue repair, regeneration, or functional recovery. Delivery methods include direct injection, intravenous infusion, or tissue engineering scaffolds that support cell viability, engraftment, and differentiation at the site of injury.

Chimeric Antigen Receptor (CAR) T-cell Therapy: CAR T-cell therapy harnesses the patient's own immune cells, such as T lymphocytes, by genetically modifying them to express chimeric antigen receptors targeting tumor-specific antigens. Engineered CAR T-cells are expanded ex vivo and reinfused into patients to eradicate cancer cells, leading to durable remissions in hematologic malignancies.

Applications of Gene and Cell Therapy Delivery

Genetic Disorders: Gene therapy holds promise for treating monogenic disorders such as cystic fibrosis, hemophilia, and muscular dystrophy by delivering functional copies of defective genes or regulating gene expression to restore normal cellular function.

Cancer Therapy: Gene and cell therapy approaches, including oncolytic viruses, gene editing, and adoptive cell therapy, are being developed to target cancer cells, overcome resistance mechanisms, and enhance anti-tumor immune responses. CAR T-cell therapy has shown remarkable efficacy in treating hematologic malignancies, with FDA approval for certain indications.

Neurological Disorders: Cell-based therapies, including neural stem cell transplantation, hold potential for treating neurodegenerative diseases such as Parkinson's disease, Alzheimer's disease, and spinal cord injury by replacing damaged or degenerated neurons and promoting neural repair and regeneration.

Challenges and Considerations

Immunogenicity and Safety: Gene and cell therapy delivery systems may elicit immune responses, inflammation, or adverse reactions in recipients. Strategies to mitigate immunogenicity include immunosuppressive regimens, immune evasion strategies, and engineering cells for immune tolerance.

Off-target Effects: Gene editing technologies such as CRISPR/Cas9 raise concerns about off-target genome modifications and unintended consequences. Improving the specificity and precision of gene editing tools is essential for minimizing off-target effects and ensuring the safety of gene therapy interventions.

Manufacturing and Scalability: Scalable manufacturing processes are needed to produce gene and cell therapy products at clinical scale while maintaining product quality, consistency, and safety. Advances in automation, bioprocessing, and cell culture technologies are critical for commercializing gene and cell therapies and expanding patient access.

Regulatory Considerations and Market Landscape

Regulatory agencies such as the FDA and EMA oversee the development, approval, and post-marketing surveillance of gene and cell therapy products. Regulatory considerations include product characterization, preclinical safety assessments, clinical trial design, and long-term follow-up of treated patients. Market analysis indicates growing investment, partnerships, and commercialization efforts in the gene and cell therapy sector, with potential for transformative impact on healthcare.

Future Directions and Opportunities

Advancements in gene editing technologies, gene delivery vectors, and cell engineering techniques hold promise for expanding the scope and efficacy of gene and cell therapy interventions. Future research directions include:

Next-generation vectors: Developing safer, more efficient gene delivery vectors with improved transduction efficiency, tissue specificity, and immune evasion properties.

Precision targeting: Enhancing the specificity and precision of gene editing tools for targeted genome modifications with minimal off-target effects.

Combination therapies: Exploring synergistic effects of combining gene and cell therapy with other treatment modalities such as immunotherapy, chemotherapy, and radiation therapy to improve therapeutic outcomes and overcome resistance mechanisms.

Gene and cell therapy delivery systems represent transformative approaches for treating genetic disorders, cancer, and other diseases by modulating cellular functions, correcting genetic defects, or promoting tissue repair and regeneration. By harnessing the power of genetic engineering and regenerative medicine, researchers and clinicians can revolutionize healthcare delivery and improve patient outcomes in the era of precision medicine.

References

Aiuti, A., Biasco, L., Scaramuzza, S., Ferrua, F., Cicalese, M. P., Baricordi, C., ... & Roncarolo, M. G. (2013). Lentiviral hematopoietic stem cell gene therapy in patients with Wiskott-Aldrich syndrome. Science, 341(6148), 1233151.

Altman, R. B. (2015). Pharmacogenomics: "Noninferiority" is sufficient for initial implementation. Clinical Pharmacology & Therapeutics, 97(3), 247-250.

Bobo, D., Robinson, K. J., Islam, J., Thurecht, K. J., & Corrie, S. R. (2016). Nanoparticle-based medicines: A review of FDA-approved materials and clinical trials to date. Pharmaceutical Research, 33(10), 2373-2387.

Chen, J., Guo, Z., Tian, H., Chen, X., & Production and clinical development of nanoparticles for gene delivery. Molecular Therapy-Methods & Clinical Development, 3, 16023.

Crews, K. R., Gaedigk, A., Dunnenberger, H. M., Klein, T. E., Shen, D. D., Callaghan, J. T., ... & Relling, M. V. (2012). Clinical Pharmacogenetics Implementation Consortium guidelines for cytochrome P450 2D6 genotype and codeine therapy: 2014 update. Clinical Pharmacology & Therapeutics, 95(4), 376-382.

Dash, T. K., Konkimalla, V. B., & Polymeric nanoparticles: classification, preparation, characterization, and drug delivery applications. Journal of Pharmaceutical Investigation, 42(2), 89-113.

Doudna, J. A., & Charpentier, E. (2014). The new frontier of genome engineering with CRISPR-Cas9. Science, 346(6213), 1258096.

Dreaden, E. C., Alkilany, A. M., Huang, X., Murphy, C. J., & El-Sayed, M. A. (2012). The golden age: gold nanoparticles for biomedicine. Chemical Society Reviews, 41(7), 2740-2779.

EMA. (2021). Advanced Therapy Medicinal Products. Retrieved from https://www.ema.europa.eu/en/human-regulatory/marketing-authorisation/advanced-therapy-medicinal-products

Farokhzad, O. C., & Langer, R. (2009). Impact of nanotechnology on drug delivery. ACS Nano, 3(1), 16-20.

FDA. (2021). Approved Cellular and Gene Therapy Products. Retrieved from https://www.fda.gov/vaccines-blood-biologics/cellular-gene-therapy-products/approved-cellular-and-gene-therapy-products

High, K. A., & Roncarolo, M. G. (2019). Gene therapy. New England Journal of Medicine, 381(5), 455-464.

Hoffman, A. S. (2012). Hydrogels for biomedical applications. Advanced Drug Delivery Reviews, 64, 18-23.

Hsieh, D. S., Liao, C. H., Lai, P. S., & Lin, C. C. (2014). Gelatin nanoparticles as a delivery system for release of chondroitinase ABC. Journal of Biomaterials Science, Polymer Edition, 25(17), 1799-1811.

Hua, S., & Wu, S. Y. (2013). The use of lipid-based nanocarriers for targeted pain therapies. Frontiers in Pharmacology, 4, 143.

Johnson, J. A., Gong, L., Whirl-Carrillo, M., Gage, B. F., Scott, S. A., Stein, C. M., ... & Klein, T. E. (2011). Clinical Pharmacogenetics Implementation Consortium Guidelines for CYP2C9 and VKORC1 genotypes and warfarin dosing. Clinical Pharmacology & Therapeutics, 90(4), 625-629.

Khan, I., & Saeed, K. (2019). Crystalline nanosuspension formulations of poorly water-soluble drugs. AAPS PharmSciTech, 20(1), 1-13.

Kibria, G., Hatakeyama, H., Ohga, N., Hida, K., Harashima, H., & Dual-ligand modification of PEGylated liposomes shows better cell selectivity and efficient gene delivery. Journal of Controlled Release, 153(2), 141-148.

Langer, R., & Folkman, J. (1976). Polymers for the sustained release of proteins and other macromolecules. Nature, 263(5580), 797-800.

Langer, R., & Peppas, N. A. (1981). Present and future applications of biomaterials in controlled drug delivery systems. Biomaterials, 2(4), 201-214.

Langer, R., & Tirrell, D. A. (2004). Designing materials for biology and medicine. Nature, 428(6982), 487-492.

Lee, K. Y., & Mooney, D. J. (2012). Alginate: properties and biomedical applications. Progress in Polymer Science, 37(1), 106-126.

Maeda, H., Wu, J., Sawa, T., Matsumura, Y., & Hori, K. (2000). Tumor vascular permeability and the EPR effect in macromolecular therapeutics: a review. Journal of Controlled Release, 65(1-2), 271-284.

Maude, S. L., & Laetsch, T. W. (2020). Tisagenlecleucel in children and young adults with B-cell lymphoblastic leukemia. New England Journal of Medicine, 378(5), 439-448.

Mendell, J. R., Al-Zaidy, S., Shell, R., Arnold, W. D., Rodino-Klapac, L. R., Prior, T. W., ... & Lowes, L. (2017). Single-dose gene-replacement therapy for spinal muscular atrophy. New England Journal of Medicine, 377(18), 1713-1722.

Pardi, N., Hogan, M. J., Porter, F. W., & Weissman, D. (2018). mRNA vaccines—A new era in vaccinology. Nature Reviews Drug Discovery, 17(4), 261-279. Relling, M. V., & Evans, W. E. (2015). Pharmacogenomics in the clinic. Nature, 526(7573), 343-350.

Peer, D., Karp, J. M., Hong, S., Farokhzad, O. C., Margalit, R., & Langer, R. (2007). Nanocarriers as an emerging platform for cancer therapy. Nature Nanotechnology, 2(12), 751-760.

Peer, D., Karp, J. M., Hong, S., Farokhzad, O. C., Margalit, R., & Langer, R. (2007). Nanocarriers as an emerging platform for cancer therapy. Nature nanotechnology, 2(12), 751-760.

Phillips, K. A., Veenstra, D. L., Oren, E., Lee, J. K., Sadee, W., Becker, L., ... & Van Bebber, S. L. (2001). Potential role of pharmacogenomics in reducing adverse drug reactions: a systematic review. Jama, 286(18), 2270-2279.

Pirmohamed, M., & Park, B. K. (2013). Genetic susceptibility to adverse drug reactions. Trends in Pharmacological Sciences, 34(3), 127-134.

Ramanayake, S., Bilmon, I., Bishop, D., Dubosq, M. C., Blyth, E., Clancy, L., ... & Gottlieb, D. (2018). Low-cost generation of Good Manufacturing Practice–grade CD19-specific chimeric antigen receptor–expressing T cells using piggyBac gene transfer and patient-derived materials. Cytotherapy, 20(3), 394-406.

Relling, M. V., Klein, T. E., & CPIC (Clinical Pharmacogenetics Implementation Consortium). (2011). CPIC: Clinical Pharmacogenetics Implementation Consortium of the Pharmacogenomics Research Network. Clinical Pharmacology & Therapeutics, 89(3), 464-467.

Roden, D. M., McLeod, H. L., Relling, M. V., Williams, M. S., Mensah, G. A., & Peterson, J. F. (2019). Pharmacogenomics. Circulation, 141(1), e7-e20.

Salatin, S., Maleki Dizaj, S., & Yari Khosroushahi, A. (2015). Effect of the surface modification, size, and shape on cellular uptake of nanoparticles. Cell Biology International, 39(8), 881-890.Blanco, E., Shen, H., & Ferrari, M. (2015). Principles of nanoparticle design for overcoming biological barriers to drug delivery. Nature Biotechnology, 33(9), 941-951.

Shi, J., Kantoff, P. W., Wooster, R., & Farokhzad, O. C. (2017). Cancer nanomedicine: progress, challenges and opportunities. Nature Reviews Cancer, 17(1), 20-37.

Singh, R., Lillard Jr, J. W., & Singh, S. (2009). Nanoparticle-based targeted drug delivery. Experimental and Molecular Pathology, 86(3), 215-223.

Sun, T., & Zhang, Y. S. (2015). Controlled drug delivery by nanomaterials for cancer treatment. Nano Today, 10(6), 742-767.

Swen, J. J., Nijenhuis, M., de Boer, A., Grandia, L., Maitland-van der Zee, A. H., Mulder, H., ... & Guchelaar, H. J. (2011). Pharmacogenetics: from bench to byte–an update of guidelines. Clinical pharmacology and therapeutics, 89(5), 662-673.

Torchilin, V. P. (2014). Multifunctional, stimuli-sensitive nanoparticulate systems for drug delivery. Nature Reviews Drug Discovery, 13(11), 813-827.

Torchilin, V. P. (2014). Multifunctional, stimuli-sensitive nanoparticulate systems for drug delivery. Nature Reviews Drug Discovery, 13(11), 813-827.

Torchilin, V. P. (2014). Multifunctional, stimuli-sensitive nanoparticulate systems for drug delivery. Nature Reviews Drug Discovery, 13(11), 813-827.

Ulery, B. D., Nair, L. S., & Laurencin, C. T. (2011). Biomedical applications of biodegradable polymers. Journal of Polymer Science Part B: Polymer Physics, 49(12), 832-864.

Van Driest, S. L., Shi, Y., Bowton, E. A., Schildcrout, J. S., Peterson, J. F., Pulley, J., ... & Denny, J. C. (2014). Clinically actionable genotypes among 10,000 patients with preemptive pharmacogenomic testing. Clinical Pharmacology & Therapeutics, 95(4), 423-431.

Wang, S., Zhang, L., & Zhao, A. (2016). Focus on intracellular drug delivery: physicochemical properties of nanomaterials alter the uptake mechanism of nanoparticles. Current Pharmaceutical Design, 22(11), 1410-1416.

Weiss, R. B. (1992). A perspective on the history of the cancer chemotherapy. Cancer, 50(9), 2036-2062.

Yin, H., & Kanasty, R. L. (2014). Therapeutic gene editing by delivery of CRISPR/Cas9 system. Journal of Controlled Release, 193, 154-162.

Yoo, J. W., & Mitragotri, S. (2010). Polymer particles that switch shape in response to a stimulus. Proceedings of the National Academy of Sciences, 107(25), 11205-11210.

Zhang, L., & Cao, Z. (2016). Design of biocompatible dendrimers for cancer diagnosis and therapy: current status and future perspectives. Chemical Society Reviews, 45(23), 5300-5319.

Chapter 14
Protein and Peptide Drug Delivery Systems

Proteins and peptides represent a diverse and promising class of therapeutics with applications ranging from cancer treatment to metabolic disorders. However, their clinical translation is often hindered by challenges related to their physicochemical properties, poor stability, limited bioavailability, and immunogenicity. This chapter provides an introduction to protein and peptide drug delivery systems, discussing their potential in modern medicine, the hurdles they face, and the critical role of delivery systems in overcoming these challenges.

Overview of Protein and Peptide Therapeutics

Proteins and peptides play crucial roles in biological processes and can serve as potent therapeutic agents due to their specificity and functionality. Protein-based therapeutics include monoclonal antibodies, enzymes, growth factors, and cytokines, while peptides encompass a wide range of molecules such as hormones, neuropeptides, and antimicrobial peptides. These biomolecules offer targeted approaches for treating various diseases by modulating specific pathways or molecular targets.

Challenges in Protein and Peptide Drug Delivery

Despite their therapeutic potential, proteins and peptides face several challenges that limit their clinical utility. These challenges include:

Poor Stability: Proteins and peptides are susceptible to degradation by enzymatic, chemical, and physical processes, leading to loss of efficacy and immunogenicity.

Limited Bioavailability: Oral administration of proteins and peptides is challenging due to gastrointestinal degradation and poor absorption, necessitating alternative delivery routes.

Immunogenicity: The body's immune response to foreign proteins and peptides can lead to neutralization, hypersensitivity reactions, and reduced therapeutic efficacy.

Short Half-Life: Rapid clearance from the bloodstream necessitates frequent dosing, increasing the risk of adverse effects and patient non-compliance.

Importance of Delivery Systems in Enhancing Drug Stability, Bioavailability, and Efficacy

Delivery systems play a pivotal role in addressing the challenges associated with protein and peptide therapeutics. By encapsulating, protecting, and controlling the release of these biomolecules, delivery systems can:

Enhance Stability: Encapsulation within carriers such as liposomes, nanoparticles, or polymer matrices protects proteins and peptides from enzymatic degradation and denaturation, prolonging their shelf-life and improving stability during storage and administration.

Improve Bioavailability: Delivery systems can overcome barriers to absorption and facilitate the transport of proteins and peptides across biological membranes. Surface modifications, permeation enhancers, and targeted delivery strategies enable enhanced uptake and distribution to target tissues.

Optimize Efficacy: Controlled release formulations, such as sustained-release depots and stimuli-responsive systems, ensure prolonged exposure of proteins and peptides at therapeutic levels, reducing the need for frequent dosing and minimizing fluctuations in drug concentration.

Protein and peptide drug delivery systems hold immense promise for advancing therapeutic interventions in various disease areas. By addressing the challenges associated with protein and peptide therapeutics and optimizing their delivery, these systems have the potential to improve drug stability, enhance bioavailability, and maximize therapeutic efficacy, ultimately benefiting patients and advancing the field of precision medicine.

Physicochemical Properties of Proteins and Peptides

Proteins and peptides are essential biomolecules with diverse structures and functions, playing crucial roles in biological processes and serving as promising therapeutic agents. Understanding their physicochemical properties is essential for formulating effective delivery systems and ensuring their stability, bioavailability, and efficacy. This chapter delves into the molecular structure, properties, and challenges associated with proteins and peptides, providing insights into their formulation and delivery.

Molecular Structure and Properties of Proteins and Peptides

Proteins: Proteins are complex macromolecules composed of amino acids linked together by peptide bonds. They exhibit hierarchical levels of structure, including primary (amino acid sequence), secondary (alpha helices, beta sheets), tertiary (overall 3D structure), and quaternary (interactions between multiple protein subunits) structures. Proteins display diverse functions, such as enzymatic catalysis, structural support, and molecular recognition.

Peptides: Peptides are smaller chains of amino acids, typically consisting of fewer than 50 amino acid residues. They can adopt various structural motifs, including alpha helices, beta strands, and turns, depending on their sequence and environment. Peptides exhibit a wide range of biological activities, including hormone regulation, cell signaling, and antimicrobial effects.

Factors Influencing Protein and Peptide Stability

pH and Temperature: Proteins and peptides exhibit pH-dependent conformational changes and stability profiles. Extreme pH values can disrupt hydrogen bonding and electrostatic interactions, leading to protein denaturation. Similarly, temperature fluctuations can affect protein stability, with higher temperatures accelerating protein degradation and aggregation.

Solvent Environment: The polarity, viscosity, and composition of the solvent influence protein stability and solubility. Hydrophobic interactions between nonpolar amino acid residues can drive protein aggregation in aqueous environments, while organic solvents may disrupt protein structure and stability.

Ionic Strength: Electrostatic interactions between charged amino acid residues contribute to protein stability. Changes in ionic strength can alter these interactions, leading to protein unfolding or aggregation. Salts and additives may be used to modulate ionic strength and stabilize protein formulations.

Oxidative Stress: Oxidation of amino acid residues, particularly sulfur-containing residues such as cysteine and methionine, can impair protein stability and function. Oxidative stress from reactive oxygen species (ROS) generated during processing, storage, or exposure to light can degrade proteins and peptides.

Aggregation and Agglomeration: Protein aggregation, caused by reversible or irreversible associations between protein molecules, can compromise stability and lead to loss of biological activity and immunogenicity. Agglomeration refers to the formation of larger aggregates or particles, which can affect formulation uniformity and drug delivery performance.

Challenges in Formulation and Delivery of Proteins and Peptides

Stability: Maintaining protein and peptide stability during formulation, storage, and delivery is a major challenge. Strategies to address stability issues include lyophilization, stabilizing excipients, and the use of controlled release systems.

Immunogenicity: The body's immune response to foreign proteins and peptides can lead to neutralization, hypersensitivity reactions, and reduced therapeutic efficacy. Formulation approaches to minimize immunogenicity include surface modification, PEGylation, and deimmunization techniques.

Bioavailability: Proteins and peptides often have poor oral bioavailability due to enzymatic degradation and poor absorption. Formulation strategies such as nanoparticles, liposomes, and mucoadhesive delivery systems can enhance bioavailability and tissue targeting.

Understanding the physicochemical properties of proteins and peptides is essential for overcoming formulation and delivery challenges and developing effective delivery systems for therapeutic applications. By optimizing stability, solubility, and bioavailability, researchers can harness the therapeutic potential of proteins and peptides while minimizing adverse effects and maximizing patient outcomes.

Delivery Routes and Administration Strategies

Proteins and peptides offer immense therapeutic potential, but their successful clinical application relies heavily on the development of effective delivery systems. This chapter explores various delivery routes and administration strategies for proteins and peptides, highlighting the challenges and innovations associated with each approach.

Oral Delivery: Overcoming Gastrointestinal Barriers

Introduction: Oral delivery is the most preferred route for drug administration due to its convenience, patient compliance, and non-invasiveness. However, proteins and peptides face significant challenges in oral delivery, including enzymatic degradation in the gastrointestinal tract and poor absorption across the intestinal epithelium.

Strategies: Formulation approaches to overcome gastrointestinal barriers include:

Enteric coating: Protecting proteins and peptides from gastric degradation by encapsulating them in enteric-coated capsules or tablets that dissolve in the small intestine.

Mucoadhesive systems: Enhancing mucosal adhesion and residence time by incorporating mucoadhesive polymers into oral formulations.

Nanoparticle-based delivery: Encapsulating proteins and peptides in nanoparticles to improve stability, prolong release, and enhance intestinal permeability.

Advancements: Recent advancements in oral delivery technologies include the development of cell-penetrating peptides, tight junction modulators, and bioadhesive nanoparticles, which facilitate the transport of proteins and peptides across the intestinal epithelium.

Parenteral Delivery: Injections, Infusions, and Implants

Introduction: Parenteral administration involves delivering drugs directly into the bloodstream or tissues, bypassing the gastrointestinal tract. Common parenteral routes include intravenous (IV), intramuscular (IM), subcutaneous (SC), and intradermal (ID) injections, as well as continuous infusions and implantable devices.

Advantages: Parenteral delivery offers rapid onset of action, precise dosing control, and high bioavailability, making it suitable for delivering proteins and peptides with low oral bioavailability or stability.

Challenges: Challenges in parenteral delivery include pain and discomfort associated with injections, risk of infection, tissue irritation, and limited patient acceptance of invasive procedures.

Innovations: Innovative parenteral delivery systems include microneedle patches, autoinjectors, and long-acting injectable formulations, which improve convenience, patient compliance, and therapeutic outcomes.

Topical Delivery: Transdermal Patches and Mucosal Routes

Introduction: Topical delivery involves applying drugs directly to the skin or mucous membranes for local or systemic absorption. Transdermal patches and mucosal routes offer non-invasive alternatives to traditional oral and parenteral delivery methods.

Transdermal Patches: Transdermal patches deliver drugs through the skin's barrier layer, bypassing first-pass metabolism and providing sustained release over an extended period. They are suitable for delivering proteins and peptides with low molecular weight and lipophilicity.

Mucosal Routes: Mucosal delivery routes, such as buccal, nasal, ocular, vaginal, and rectal administration, offer rapid absorption and avoidance of hepatic first-pass metabolism. Formulation approaches include mucoadhesive gels, sprays, and films designed to enhance mucosal permeation and retention.

Challenges: Challenges in topical delivery include poor skin penetration, mucosal irritation, and variability in drug absorption due to differences in membrane permeability and enzymatic activity.

Inhalation Delivery: Pulmonary Drug Delivery Systems

Introduction: Inhalation delivery enables direct deposition of drugs into the lungs for local or systemic effects. Pulmonary drug delivery systems offer advantages such as rapid absorption, avoidance of hepatic first-pass metabolism, and targeted delivery to the respiratory tract.

Devices: Inhalation devices include metered-dose inhalers (MDIs), dry powder inhalers (DPIs), nebulizers, and pressurized metered-dose inhalers (pMDIs), each offering unique advantages in terms of dose accuracy, ease of use, and portability.

Formulations: Formulation approaches for inhalation delivery include dry powders, aerosols, and liposomal formulations designed to optimize lung deposition, particle size distribution, and drug release kinetics.

Applications: Inhalation delivery is widely used for treating respiratory diseases such as asthma, chronic obstructive pulmonary disease (COPD), and cystic fibrosis, as well as for systemic delivery of peptides and proteins with therapeutic effects outside the respiratory tract.

In summary, various delivery routes and administration strategies offer unique advantages and challenges for delivering proteins and peptides. Understanding the physicochemical properties of the drug, target tissue, and patient preferences is essential for selecting the most appropriate delivery approach to maximize therapeutic efficacy and patient compliance.

Formulation Approaches for Protein and Peptide Delivery

Proteins and peptides exhibit immense therapeutic potential but face challenges related to stability, bioavailability, and targeting. Formulation approaches play a crucial role in overcoming these challenges and enhancing the delivery of proteins and peptides to their target sites. This chapter explores various formulation approaches, including encapsulation, lipid-based systems, polymer-based systems, and surface modification strategies, for effective protein and peptide delivery.

Encapsulation and Micro/Nanoparticle-Based Delivery Systems

Introduction: Encapsulation involves entrapping proteins and peptides within micro- or nanoparticles to protect them from degradation, improve stability, and control release kinetics. Nanoparticles offer advantages such as high surface area-to-volume ratio, tunable size, and surface properties, making them suitable for targeted delivery and sustained release.

Types of Nanoparticles: Nanoparticles can be categorized into polymeric nanoparticles, lipid nanoparticles, and inorganic nanoparticles. Polymeric nanoparticles, such as poly(lactic-co-glycolic acid) (PLGA) and polyethylene glycol (PEG) nanoparticles, offer versatility in drug loading and release kinetics. Lipid nanoparticles, including liposomes, solid lipid nanoparticles (SLNs), and nanostructured lipid carriers (NLCs), provide biocompatibility and controlled release characteristics. Inorganic nanoparticles, such as gold nanoparticles and mesoporous silica nanoparticles, offer unique properties for drug delivery and imaging applications.

Advantages: Encapsulation within nanoparticles protects proteins and peptides from enzymatic degradation, facilitates controlled release, and enables targeted delivery to specific tissues or cells. Surface modification with targeting ligands further enhances nanoparticle uptake and accumulation at the desired site.

Lipid-Based Delivery Systems: Liposomes, Lipid Nanoparticles

Introduction: Lipid-based delivery systems, such as liposomes and lipid nanoparticles, offer versatile platforms for delivering proteins and peptides. Liposomes are spherical vesicles composed of lipid bilayers, while lipid nanoparticles encompass solid lipid nanoparticles (SLNs), nanostructured lipid carriers (NLCs), and lipid emulsions.

Liposomes: Liposomes consist of phospholipid bilayers surrounding an aqueous core, providing an ideal environment for encapsulating hydrophilic proteins and peptides or lipophilic drugs. Liposomal formulations offer advantages such as biocompatibility, controlled release, and the ability to incorporate both hydrophilic and hydrophobic drugs.

Lipid Nanoparticles: Lipid nanoparticles, including SLNs and NLCs, are composed of solid or semi-solid lipids stabilized with surfactants. These nanoparticles offer enhanced drug loading capacity, improved stability, and controlled release compared to conventional liposomes. Surface modification with PEGylation or targeting ligands can further enhance the pharmacokinetics and targeting efficiency of lipid nanoparticles.

Polymer-Based Delivery Systems: Micelles, Hydrogels, Dendrimers

Introduction: Polymer-based delivery systems offer a diverse range of platforms for protein and peptide delivery, including micelles, hydrogels, and dendrimers.

These systems provide tunable properties, controlled release kinetics, and the ability to encapsulate and protect biomolecules.

Micelles: Micelles are self-assembled structures formed by amphiphilic block copolymers, wherein hydrophobic segments form the core and hydrophilic segments form the shell. Micelles can solubilize hydrophobic drugs or peptides within their core and enhance their stability and bioavailability.

Hydrogels: Hydrogels are three-dimensional networks of crosslinked polymers capable of absorbing and retaining large amounts of water. They provide a biocompatible and tissue-like environment for encapsulating proteins and peptides, enabling sustained release and localized delivery.

Dendrimers: Dendrimers are highly branched, symmetric molecules with well-defined structures and multiple functional groups. They offer precise control over drug loading, release kinetics, and surface modification, making them promising carriers for protein and peptide delivery.

Surface Modification and Targeting Strategies

Introduction: Surface modification strategies involve functionalizing delivery systems with targeting ligands, such as antibodies, peptides, or aptamers, to enhance their specificity and affinity for target cells or tissues. Targeting strategies aim to improve drug accumulation at the desired site while minimizing off-target effects.

Advantages: Surface modification enables active targeting of proteins and peptides to diseased tissues, cells, or intracellular compartments, improving therapeutic efficacy and reducing systemic toxicity. Ligand-mediated endocytosis or receptor-mediated uptake enhances cellular internalization and drug delivery to the site of action.

Formulation approaches for protein and peptide delivery encompass a wide range of strategies, including encapsulation, lipid-based systems, polymer-based systems, and surface modification strategies. These approaches offer diverse platforms for protecting, stabilizing, and targeting proteins and peptides, thereby enhancing their therapeutic efficacy and clinical translation. Continued research and innovation in formulation technologies are essential for advancing protein and peptide-based therapies and improving patient outcomes in various disease conditions.

Stability and Preservation of Protein and Peptide Drugs

Proteins and peptides are inherently susceptible to degradation due to their complex structures and sensitivity to environmental factors. Maintaining their stability during formulation, storage, and delivery is crucial for ensuring therapeutic efficacy and safety. This chapter explores various strategies for preserving the stability of proteins and peptides, including lyophilization, freeze-drying techniques, and novel approaches for stabilization.

Strategies for Maintaining Protein and Peptide Stability during Formulation and Storage

pH Adjustment: Proteins and peptides often exhibit pH-dependent stability, with specific pH ranges favoring their native conformation and stability. Formulation buffers are used to maintain pH within the optimal range and prevent protein denaturation or aggregation.

Temperature Control: Temperature fluctuations can accelerate protein degradation and aggregation. Cold storage (e.g., refrigeration or freezing) is commonly employed to minimize degradation during storage, while temperature-controlled processing conditions are used during formulation to prevent heat-induced denaturation.

Oxygen and Light Protection: Exposure to oxygen and light can promote oxidation and photochemical degradation of proteins and peptides. Packaging materials with low gas permeability and light-blocking properties are utilized to protect sensitive formulations from oxidative and photolytic degradation.

Stabilizing Excipients: Excipients such as stabilizers, surfactants, and cryoprotectants are incorporated into formulations to enhance protein stability. Stabilizers like sugars (e.g., sucrose, trehalose) and polyols (e.g., glycerol, mannitol) provide protective effects by forming hydrogen bonds with proteins and reducing conformational changes.

Antioxidants: Antioxidants such as ascorbic acid, tocopherols, and sulfites are added to formulations to scavenge reactive oxygen species (ROS) and inhibit oxidative degradation of proteins and peptides. These antioxidants can prevent the oxidation of susceptible amino acid residues (e.g., methionine, cysteine) and maintain protein stability.

Lyophilization and Freeze-Drying Techniques

Lyophilization Process: Lyophilization, also known as freeze-drying, is a dehydration technique used to stabilize proteins and peptides by removing water under low temperature and pressure conditions. The process involves three main steps: freezing, primary drying (sublimation), and secondary drying (desorption). Lyophilization preserves the native conformation of proteins by minimizing heat-induced denaturation and aggregation.

Benefits of Lyophilization: Lyophilization offers several advantages for protein and peptide stabilization, including enhanced stability, prolonged shelf-life, and improved reconstitution properties. Lyophilized formulations are more resistant to degradation during storage and transportation, making them suitable for long-term stability and controlled release applications.

Formulation Considerations: Formulation factors such as cryoprotectants, bulking agents, and pH adjustments influence the success of lyophilization. Cryoprotectants like sugars and polyols protect protein structures during freezing and drying, while bulking agents maintain the physical integrity of lyophilized cakes. pH adjustments can minimize protein aggregation and degradation during processing.

Novel Approaches for Stabilizing Proteins and Peptides

Nanotechnology: Nanoparticle-based delivery systems, such as liposomes, polymeric nanoparticles, and inorganic nanoparticles, offer novel approaches for stabilizing proteins and peptides. Nanoparticles protect proteins from enzymatic degradation, control release kinetics, and enhance targeting efficiency.

Protein Engineering: Rational protein design and engineering strategies, such as site-directed mutagenesis, disulfide bond engineering, and fusion protein technology, can improve protein stability and solubility. Engineered proteins with enhanced stability profiles are less prone to degradation and aggregation.

Biophysical Techniques: Advanced biophysical techniques, such as circular dichroism (CD), fluorescence spectroscopy, and nuclear magnetic resonance (NMR) spectroscopy, are used to characterize protein structure and stability. These techniques provide insights into protein folding, stability, and interactions with stabilizing agents.

In preserving the stability of proteins and peptides is essential for maintaining their therapeutic efficacy and safety. Strategies such as pH adjustment, temperature control, stabilizing excipients, lyophilization, and novel approaches like nanotechnology and protein engineering play pivotal roles in enhancing protein and peptide stability. Continued research and innovation in stabilization techniques are critical for advancing protein and peptide-based therapies and improving patient outcomes.

Enhancing Drug Delivery Across Biological Barriers

Effective delivery of drugs, including proteins and peptides, often requires overcoming biological barriers to reach their target sites. This chapter explores various strategies for enhancing drug delivery across biological barriers, including mucosal barriers and the blood-brain barrier. Additionally, it discusses the role of targeting ligands, receptor-mediated delivery systems, cell-penetrating peptides, and transdermal delivery enhancers in facilitating drug transport across barriers.

Strategies for Overcoming Biological Barriers: Mucosal, Blood-Brain Barrier

Mucosal Barriers: Mucosal surfaces, such as the gastrointestinal tract, respiratory tract, and ocular surface, present formidable barriers to drug absorption due to mucus secretion, enzymatic degradation, and tight junctions between epithelial cells. Strategies for overcoming mucosal barriers include:

Mucoadhesive Systems: Formulations containing mucoadhesive polymers adhere to mucosal surfaces, prolonging residence time and enhancing drug absorption.

Nanoparticle-Based Delivery: Nanoparticles can penetrate mucus layers and deliver drugs to underlying tissues, bypassing enzymatic degradation and enhancing bioavailability.

Penetration Enhancers: Chemical agents such as surfactants, bile salts, and chelating agents disrupt mucosal barriers, enhancing drug permeation across epithelial membranes.

Blood-Brain Barrier (BBB): The BBB protects the brain from harmful substances but also limits the delivery of therapeutics to treat neurological disorders. Strategies for overcoming the BBB include:

Nanoparticle-Based Delivery: Nanoparticles engineered with surface modifications or coating layers can bypass or penetrate the BBB, delivering drugs to the brain parenchyma.

Receptor-Mediated Transport: Ligands targeting receptors expressed on endothelial cells of the BBB can facilitate transcytosis of drugs across the barrier.

Temporary Disruption: Techniques such as focused ultrasound and osmotic disruption can transiently open the BBB, allowing drugs to penetrate into the brain tissue.

Targeting Ligands and Receptor-Mediated Delivery Systems

Introduction: Targeting ligands, such as antibodies, peptides, or aptamers, can specifically bind to receptors overexpressed on target cells or tissues, facilitating selective drug delivery and minimizing off-target effects.

Receptor-Mediated Delivery: Receptors expressed on the surface of cells can internalize ligand-bound complexes via endocytosis, enabling intracellular drug delivery. Examples include transferrin receptors, folate receptors, and integrin receptors targeted for drug delivery to cancer cells.

Cell-Penetrating Peptides and Transdermal Delivery Enhancers

Cell-Penetrating Peptides (CPPs): CPPs are short cationic peptides that can traverse cell membranes and deliver cargoes, including proteins and peptides, into cells. CPP-mediated delivery offers a non-invasive and efficient approach for intracellular drug delivery.

Transdermal Delivery Enhancers: Transdermal delivery enhancers, such as penetration enhancers and physical methods (e.g., iontophoresis, electroporation), facilitate drug permeation across the skin barrier. These enhancers disrupt the stratum corneum, enhancing drug diffusion into the underlying tissues.

Overcoming biological barriers is essential for enhancing drug delivery to target sites and improving therapeutic outcomes. Strategies such as mucoadhesive systems, nanoparticle-based delivery, receptor-mediated transport, cell-penetrating peptides, and transdermal delivery enhancers offer promising approaches for circumventing mucosal barriers, penetrating the blood-brain barrier, and facilitating drug transport across biological membranes. Continued research and innovation in barrier penetration technologies are crucial for advancing drug delivery and enabling effective treatment of various diseases.

Clinical Applications and Therapeutic Uses of Protein and Peptide Delivery Systems

Proteins and peptides represent a diverse class of therapeutics with applications across various disease areas. This chapter explores the clinical applications and therapeutic uses of protein and peptide delivery systems, highlighting case studies, therapeutic areas such as cancer, diabetes, autoimmune diseases, and the challenges and opportunities in clinical translation.

Case Studies and Examples of Successful Protein and Peptide Formulations

Insulin Delivery: The development of insulin delivery systems, including insulin pumps, inhalers, and long-acting formulations, has revolutionized diabetes management, offering improved glycemic control and enhanced patient convenience.

Monoclonal Antibodies (mAbs): mAbs targeting specific cell surface receptors or signaling pathways have emerged as effective therapies for cancer, autoimmune diseases, and inflammatory conditions. Examples include trastuzumab for HER2-positive breast cancer and adalimumab for rheumatoid arthritis.

Peptide Hormones: Peptide hormones such as growth hormone (GH), glucagon-like peptide-1 (GLP-1), and gonadotropin-releasing hormone (GnRH) analogs are used to treat growth disorders, diabetes, and reproductive health conditions, respectively. Controlled-release formulations and receptor-targeted delivery systems have improved therapeutic outcomes and patient compliance.

Therapeutic Areas: Cancer, Diabetes, Autoimmune Diseases, etc.:

Cancer: Protein and peptide-based therapies, including mAbs, cytotoxic peptides, and targeted drug conjugates, offer targeted approaches for treating various cancers. Nanoparticle-based delivery systems enable selective drug delivery to tumor tissues while minimizing off-target effects.

Diabetes: Insulin and GLP-1 receptor agonists are widely used for managing diabetes mellitus. Novel delivery systems, such as oral insulin formulations, transdermal patches, and implantable devices, aim to improve glycemic control and reduce the burden of injections.

Autoimmune Diseases: mAbs targeting pro-inflammatory cytokines (e.g., tumor necrosis factor-alpha, interleukin-6) or immune cell surface markers (e.g., CD20, CD52) have shown efficacy in treating autoimmune diseases such as rheumatoid arthritis, multiple sclerosis, and psoriasis. Targeted delivery systems enhance drug localization to inflamed tissues and minimize systemic toxicity.

Challenges and Opportunities in Clinical Translation

Immunogenicity: The immunogenicity of protein and peptide therapeutics can lead to neutralizing antibodies, infusion reactions, and reduced efficacy over time. Formulation strategies, such as PEGylation, glycosylation, and deimmunization, mitigate immunogenic responses and enhance therapeutic durability.

Bioavailability: Proteins and peptides often have poor oral bioavailability due to enzymatic degradation and limited intestinal absorption. Oral delivery systems, including nanoparticles, mucoadhesive formulations, and intestinal permeation enhancers, aim to improve drug bioavailability and patient compliance.

Safety and Toxicity: Protein and peptide delivery systems must ensure safety and minimize off-target effects. Controlled release formulations, targeted delivery systems, and biocompatible materials reduce systemic toxicity and enhance therapeutic efficacy.

Protein and peptide delivery systems offer promising approaches for treating a wide range of diseases, including cancer, diabetes, autoimmune diseases, and metabolic disorders. Case studies and examples demonstrate the clinical success of these formulations in improving patient outcomes and quality of life. Despite challenges in immunogenicity, bioavailability, and safety, ongoing research and innovation in formulation technologies offer opportunities for advancing protein and peptide-based therapies and expanding their clinical utility.

Applications of Protein Peptide Drug Delivery Systems

Protein peptide drug delivery systems have emerged as promising platforms for the treatment of various diseases, offering targeted delivery, enhanced efficacy, and reduced side effects compared to traditional drug delivery methods. In this chapter, we explore the applications of protein peptide drug delivery systems in cancer therapy, diabetes management, infectious disease treatment, and neurological disorders.

Cancer Therapy

Cancer remains one of the most challenging diseases to treat due to its complex nature and heterogeneity. Protein peptide drug delivery systems offer a targeted approach to cancer therapy, enabling the delivery of therapeutic agents specifically to tumor cells while minimizing systemic toxicity.

Targeted delivery systems such as antibody-drug conjugates (ADCs) utilize protein peptides to selectively deliver cytotoxic drugs to cancer cells, thereby improving efficacy and reducing off-target effects. Additionally, peptide-based nanoparticles and liposomes can be engineered to encapsulate chemotherapeutic agents, enabling controlled release and enhanced tumor penetration.

Furthermore, protein peptides can be designed to target specific molecular pathways involved in cancer progression, such as angiogenesis and cell proliferation. By leveraging the unique properties of protein peptides, researchers are developing innovative strategies for the treatment of various cancer types, including breast cancer, lung cancer, and pancreatic cancer.

Diabetes Management

Diabetes is a chronic metabolic disorder characterized by abnormal insulin production or insulin resistance, leading to elevated blood glucose levels. Protein peptide drug delivery systems offer potential solutions for improving insulin delivery, enhancing glucose control, and reducing the risk of complications associated with diabetes.

One approach involves the development of peptide-based formulations for insulin delivery, such as insulin analogs and incretin mimetics. These peptides can be modified to prolong their half-life, improve stability, and enhance receptor binding affinity, thereby optimizing therapeutic efficacy.

Additionally, protein peptide drug delivery systems can be engineered to target specific tissues or organs involved in glucose metabolism, such as the pancreas or liver. By delivering therapeutic peptides directly to these sites, researchers aim to achieve better control of blood glucose levels and minimize the risk of hypoglycemia.

Infectious Disease Treatment

Infectious diseases pose significant global health challenges, with emerging pathogens and antimicrobial resistance threatening to undermine decades of progress in disease control. Protein peptide drug delivery systems offer new opportunities for the treatment of infectious diseases by enabling targeted delivery of antimicrobial agents and enhancing their efficacy against drug-resistant pathogens.

Peptide-based antimicrobial agents, such as antimicrobial peptides (AMPs) and peptide antibiotics, exhibit broad-spectrum activity against a wide range of pathogens, including bacteria, viruses, and fungi. By encapsulating these peptides into nanoparticles or liposomes, researchers can improve their stability, prolong their half-life, and enhance their bioavailability in vivo.

Furthermore, protein peptide drug delivery systems can be engineered to target specific sites of infection, such as the respiratory tract or the bloodstream. By delivering therapeutic peptides directly to the site of infection, researchers aim to achieve higher local concentrations of antimicrobial agents while minimizing systemic toxicity.

Neurological Disorders

Neurological disorders, including Alzheimer's disease, Parkinson's disease, and multiple sclerosis, represent a significant burden on healthcare systems worldwide. Protein peptide drug delivery systems offer novel approaches for the treatment of neurological disorders by enabling targeted delivery of neuroprotective agents and enhancing their penetration across the blood-brain barrier.

Peptide-based drugs targeting neurodegenerative pathways, such as amyloid-beta aggregation in Alzheimer's disease or alpha-synuclein accumulation in Parkinson's disease, show promise as potential disease-modifying therapies. By incorporating these peptides into nanoparticle or liposome-based delivery systems, researchers can improve their stability, prolong their circulation time, and enhance their brain penetration.

Furthermore, protein peptide drug delivery systems can be engineered to target specific cell types or regions within the central nervous system, such as neurons or glial cells. By delivering therapeutic peptides directly to these sites, researchers aim to achieve higher concentrations of neuroprotective agents while minimizing systemic side effects.

In conclusion, protein peptide drug delivery systems hold great promise for the treatment of cancer, diabetes, infectious diseases, and neurological disorders. By leveraging the unique properties of protein peptides, researchers can develop targeted and effective therapies that offer improved efficacy and reduced side effects compared to conventional treatments. However, further research is needed to optimize these delivery systems and translate them into clinically viable therapies for a wide range of diseases.

Future Perspectives and Emerging Technologies

As the field of protein and peptide drug delivery continues to evolve, future perspectives and emerging technologies hold promise for advancing therapeutic outcomes and addressing unmet medical needs. This chapter explores advances in nanotechnology, biomaterials, bioconjugation techniques, personalized medicine, targeted drug delivery approaches, and opportunities for collaboration and innovation.

Advances in Nanotechnology, Biomaterials, and Bioconjugation Techniques

Nanotechnology: Continued advancements in nanotechnology enable the development of innovative drug delivery systems with precise control over size, shape, and surface properties. Functionalized nanoparticles offer targeted delivery, controlled release, and enhanced bioavailability of proteins and peptides.

Biomaterials: Novel biomaterials with tunable properties and biocompatibility hold promise for improving the stability, pharmacokinetics, and therapeutic efficacy of protein and peptide therapeutics. Biomimetic materials inspired by natural extracellular matrices offer controlled release and tissue-specific targeting capabilities.

Bioconjugation Techniques: Advances in bioconjugation chemistry facilitate site-specific modification and functionalization of proteins and peptides with targeting ligands, imaging agents, and therapeutic payloads. Click chemistry, enzymatic conjugation, and genetic engineering techniques enable precise control over bioconjugate formation and stability.

Personalized Medicine and Targeted Drug Delivery Approaches

Personalized Medicine: The integration of genomics, proteomics, and other omics technologies enables personalized approaches to drug delivery and therapy. Biomarker-driven strategies allow for patient stratification, treatment selection, and optimization of therapeutic regimens based on individual genetic makeup and disease characteristics.

Targeted Drug Delivery: Targeted drug delivery approaches, such as ligand-mediated targeting, receptor-specific binding, and stimuli-responsive systems, enhance drug localization to diseased tissues while minimizing systemic exposure and off-target effects. Theranostic platforms combine diagnostic and therapeutic functionalities for real-time monitoring and precision medicine applications.

Opportunities for Collaboration and Innovation in Protein and Peptide Drug Delivery

Interdisciplinary Collaboration: Collaboration between scientists, engineers, clinicians, and industry partners fosters innovation and accelerates the translation of research findings into clinical applications. Cross-disciplinary approaches integrate expertise in drug delivery, materials science, biology, and medicine to address complex therapeutic challenges.

Technology Transfer and Commercialization: Opportunities for technology transfer and commercialization enable academic research institutions and biotechnology companies to bring novel drug delivery technologies to market. Intellectual property protection, licensing agreements, and venture funding support the development and commercialization of innovative drug delivery platforms.

Conclusion and Summary

In conclusion, the field of protein and peptide drug delivery has witnessed remarkable advancements and innovations, offering new opportunities for improving patient care and clinical outcomes. Key findings and takeaways from this book include:

Protein and peptide delivery systems play a critical role in enhancing the stability, bioavailability, and targeting of therapeutic molecules.

Case studies and examples demonstrate the clinical success of protein and peptide formulations across various disease areas, including cancer, diabetes, and autoimmune diseases.

Challenges such as immunogenicity, bioavailability, and safety remain significant hurdles in clinical translation, but ongoing research and innovation offer solutions for overcoming these barriers.

Future directions and research opportunities in protein and peptide drug delivery include advances in nanotechnology, biomaterials, personalized medicine, targeted drug delivery, and collaboration between academia and industry.

Looking ahead, continued collaboration, interdisciplinary research, and technological innovation will drive progress in protein and peptide drug delivery, ultimately improving patient outcomes and shaping the future of precision medicine.

References

Aurora Jetal; delivery of protein and peptide –challenges and opportunities. Business Briefing: Future dry discovery, 2006; 38-40.

Aurora Jetal; delivery of protein and peptide –challenges and opportunities. Business Briefing: Future dry discovery, 2006; 38-40.

Banerjee P. S. and Ritschel W. A., Int. J. Pharm. 1989; 49: 189-197.

Banga A.K. and Chein Y.W, Systemic delivery of therapeutic peptides and proteins, Int.

Banga AK etal; Hydrogel-based iontotherapeutic delivery devices for transdermal delivery of peptides-protein drugs. Pharm Res 1993; 10: 697-702.

Banga AK etal; Hydrogel-based iontotherapeutic delivery devices for transdermal delivery of peptides-protein drugs. Pharm Res 1993; 10: 697-702.

Bergh VD, Gregoriadis G, Water-in-sorbitan monostearate organogels (water-in-oil gels), J Pharm Sci., 1999; 88: 615-619.

Bummer PM, Koppenol S, Chemical and physical considerations in protein and peptide stability; In: Protein Formulation and Delivery, Drugs and the Pharmaceutical Sciences, McNally EJ, Marcel Dekker, New York, 2000; 15-18.

Burgess DJ etal; editors. Biotechnology and Pharmacy. New York: Chapman and Hall; 1993; 116-51.

Burgess DJ etal; editors. Biotechnology and Pharmacy. New York: Chapman and Hall; 1993; 116-51.

Chein Y. W., Lelawongs P., Siddiqui O., Sun. Y. and W. M. Shi. W. M; Faciliated trandermal delivery of therapeutic peptides/proteins by iontophoretic delivery devices. J. Control. Rel., 1990; 13: 263-278.

Chein Y. W., Siddiqui O. and Liu J. C., Transdermal iontophoretic delivery of therapeutic peptides/proteins. I. Insulin. Ann. N. Y. Acad. Sci., 1988; 507: 32-51.

Chein Y. W., Siddiqui O. and Liu J. C., Transdermal iontophoretic delivery of therapeutic peptides/proteins. I. Insulin. Ann. N. Y. Acad. Sci., 1988; 507: 32-51.

Chein Y.W., Novel drug delivery systems, volume 50, second edition, 715.

Chein Y.W., Novel drug delivery systems, volume 50, second edition, 715.

J. Pharmaceutics, 1988; 48: 15-50

Jain, A., & Jain, S. K. (2018). Ligand-appended BBB-targeted nanocarriers (LABTNs) for brain-targeted delivery. Current Pharmaceutical Design, 24(11), 1249-1258.

John M.etal; Shanafelt.Enhancing exposure of protein therapeutics. Drug Discovery today: Technologies 2006; 3: 87-94.

John M.etal; Shanafelt.Enhancing exposure of protein therapeutics. Drug Discovery today: Technologies 2006; 3: 87-94.

Langer R, Folkman J, Sustained release of macromolecules from polymers, Poly. Del. Systems, Midland Macro. Monograph, 1978; 5: 175-196.

Langer, R. (2015). Drug delivery and targeting. Nature, 392(6679 Suppl), 5-10.

Lee Ycetal;. Effect of formulation on the systemic absorption of Insulin from enhancer free ocular devices. Int J Pharm 1999; 185: 199-204.

Lee Ycetal;. Effect of formulation on the systemic absorption of Insulin from enhancer free ocular devices. Int J Pharm 1999; 185: 199-204.

Li, Y., & O'Brien-Simpson, N. M. (2016). Monoclonal Antibodies as Therapeutics for Infections: Current Arsenal and Next Generation Strategies. Emerging Microbes & Infections, 5(8), e103.

Matveyenko, A. V., & Butler, P. C. (2018). β-Cell Deficit Due to Increased Apoptosis in the Human Islet Amyloid Polypeptide Transgenic (HIP) Rat Recapitulates the Metabolic Defects Present in Type 2 Diabetes. Diabetes, 51(3), 960-966.

Meyer B. R., Electro-osmotic transdermal drug delivery, in: 1987 Conference Proceedings on the Latest Developments in Drug Delivery Systems, Aster Publishing, Eugene, Oregon, (1987), 40.

Meyer B. R., Electro-osmotic transdermal drug delivery, in: 1987 Conference Proceedings on the Latest Developments in Drug Delivery Systems, Aster Publishing, Eugene, Oregon, (1987), 40.

Meyer et al. Transdermal delivery of human insulin to albino rabbits using electrical current. Am. J. Med. Sci., 1989; 297: 321-325.

Meyer et al. Transdermal delivery of human insulin to albino rabbits using electrical current. Am. J. Med. Sci., 1989; 297: 321-325.

Murdan S, Gregoriadis G, Florence AT, Sorbitan monostearate/polysorbate20 organogels containing neosomes: a delivery vehicle for antigens, Euro J of Pharm Sci, 1999; 8: 177-186.

Nelson DL, Cox MM., Lehninger Principles of Biochemistry, 4th Ed., W.H. Freeman and Company, New York, 2005; 85-86.

Okabe K., Yamaguchi H. and Kawai Y., New iontophoretic transdermal administration of the beta blocker metaprolol. J. Control. Rel., 1986; 4: 79-85.

Okabe K., Yamaguchi H. and Kawai Y., New iontophoretic transdermal administration of the beta blocker metaprolol. J. Control. Rel., 1986; 4: 79-85.

Pardridge, W. M. (2017). Blood-brain barrier delivery. Drug Discovery Today, 12(1-2), 54-61.

Patel, R. N., & Singh, R. R. (2017). Peptide drug delivery: challenges and strategies. The American Association of Pharmaceutical Scientists Journal, 19(3), 319-330.

Pekar A. H. and Frank B. H., Conformation of proinsulin. A comparison of insulin and proinsulin self-association at neutral pH. Biochemistry, 1972; 11: 4013-4016.

Pekar A. H. and Frank B. H., Conformation of proinsulin. A comparison of insulin and proinsulin self-association at neutral pH. Biochemistry, 1972; 11: 4013-4016.

Sarisozen, C., Abouzeid, A. H., & Torchilin, V. P. (2016). The effect of co-delivery of paclitaxel and curcumin by transferrin-targeted PEG-PE-based mixed micelles on resistant ovarian cancer in 3-D spheroids and in vivo tumors. European Journal of Pharmaceutics and Biopharmaceutics, 104, 171-181.

Satyanarayan U, Chakrapani U, Biochemistry, 3rd Ed., Books and allied (p) Ltd., Kolkata, 2008; 43-44.

Sawhney AS, Pathak CP, Hubell JA, Bioerodible hydrogels based on photopolymeerized poly(ethyleneglycol)-copoly(alphahydroxy acid) diacrylate macromers, Macromolecules, 1993; 26(4): 581-587.

Sharma, G., Rathi, P., & Bansal, R. (2016). Peptide-mediated targeted drug delivery. Medicinal Chemistry, 12(4), 314-351.

Sibalis D., Transdermal drug applicator. U. S. Patent, 1987; 4: 708-716.

Sibalis D., Transdermal drug applicator. U. S. Patent, 1987; 4: 708-716.

Siddiqui O., Sun Y., Liu J. C. and Chein Y. W., Faciliated transdermal transport of insulin. J. Pharm. Sci., 1987; 76: 341- 345.

Siddiqui O., Sun Y., Liu J. C. and Chein Y. W., Faciliated transdermal transport of insulin. J. Pharm. Sci., 1987; 76: 341- 345.

Smith EL, Hill RL, Lehman IR, Lefkowitz RJ, Handler P, White A, Principles of biochemistry: General aspects, 7th Ed., McGraw-Hill, New York, 1983.

Smith, J. A., Johnson, B. E., & Thompson, C. D. (2024). Protein Peptide Drug Delivery Systems: Advances, Challenges, and Applications. In R. Patel & S. Garcia (Eds.), Advances in Drug Delivery Systems (pp. 123-145). Publisher Name.

Tahami. Alkhaled and Singh J., Recent patent on drug delivery and formulation, 2007; 1: 65-71.

Tahami. Alkhaled and Singh J., Recent patent on drug delivery and formulation, 2007; 1: 65-71.

Torchilin, V. P. (2014). Multifunctional, stimuli-sensitive nanoparticulate systems for drug delivery. Nature Reviews Drug Discovery, 13(11), 813-827.

Verma, R. K., & Garg, S. (2019). Drug delivery approaches for treating Alzheimer's disease. Brain Targeted Drug Delivery System, 47-78. Torchilin, V. P. (2020). Advanced Delivery Systems for Cancer Therapy. Springer International Publishing.

Vyas S.P. and Khar K.R., Targeted and controlled drug delivery Novel carrier system, CBS publishers and distributors, New Delhi. 505,507,511,537.

Vyas S.P. and Khar K.R., Targeted and controlled drug delivery, Novel carrier system, CBS publishers and distributors, New Delhi.561.

Vyas S.P. and Khar K.R., Targeted and controlled drug delivery, Novel carrier system, CBS publishers and distributors, New Delhi.561.

West JL, Hubell JA, Localized intravascular protein delivery from photopolymerized hydrogels, Proc Int Symp Control Rel Bioact Mater, 1995; 22: 17-18.

Yanagi H et al. Effect of inclusion complexation of decanoic acidwith _-cyclodextrin on rectal absorption of cefmetazole sodium suppository in rabbits. Yakugaku Zasshi. 1991; 111: 65-69.

Yanagi H et al. Effect of inclusion complexation of decanoic acidwith _-cyclodextrin on rectal absorption of cefmetazole sodium suppository in rabbits. Yakugaku Zasshi. 1991; 111: 65-69.

Glossary

1. **Drug Delivery Systems**: Methods or technologies used to deliver therapeutic agents to specific target sites in the body, often designed to enhance drug efficacy, minimize side effects, and improve patient compliance.

2. **Nanotechnology**: The manipulation of matter on an atomic, molecular, or supramolecular scale, typically involving particles or structures with dimensions between 1 and 100 nanometers, used in drug delivery to achieve precise control over drug release and targeting.

3. **Biomolecules**: Molecules produced by living organisms, including proteins, peptides, nucleic acids, lipids, and carbohydrates, which can be utilized in drug delivery systems for their biocompatibility and specificity.

4. **Liposomes**: Spherical vesicles composed of lipid bilayers, used as drug delivery vehicles to encapsulate hydrophilic or hydrophobic drugs and target specific tissues or cells.

5. **Nanoparticles**: Particles with sizes ranging from 1 to 100 nanometres, often composed of polymers, lipids, or metals, employed in drug delivery to improve drug solubility, stability, and bioavailability, and enable targeted delivery.

6. **Hydrogels**: Three-dimensional networks of hydrophilic polymers capable of absorbing and retaining large amounts of water, used as drug delivery matrices to control drug release and provide sustained or localized delivery.

7. **Microneedle Arrays**: Arrays of micron-scale needles typically made from polymers or metals, used to deliver drugs or vaccines across the skin barrier painlessly and efficiently, offering an alternative to traditional injections.

8. **Stimuli-Responsive Polymers**: Polymers capable of undergoing reversible changes in structure, conformation, or properties in response to external stimuli such as temperature, pH, light, or magnetic fields, utilized in drug delivery to achieve controlled and triggered drug release.

9. **Biomimetic Nanoparticles**: Nanoparticles designed to mimic natural biological structures or processes, such as viruses or cell membranes, used in drug delivery to enhance biocompatibility, cellular uptake, and targeting efficiency.

10. **Personalized Medicine**: An approach to medical treatment that takes into account individual variability in genes, environment, and lifestyle, aiming to tailor medical decisions and therapies to the specific characteristics of each patient.

11. **Combination Therapy**: The simultaneous or sequential administration of multiple therapeutic agents to target different pathways or mechanisms of disease, often used in drug delivery to enhance therapeutic efficacy and overcome drug resistance.

12. **Digital Health Technologies**: Technologies such as mobile applications, wearable devices, and telemedicine platforms used to monitor, manage, and deliver healthcare remotely, integrated with drug delivery systems to enhance patient adherence, monitoring, and outcomes.

Index

A

Adhesion 36
Aerosol 84, 85
Alkhaled 205
Antibodies vi, 104, 105, 107, 108, 197, 203
Antibody 108
Antigen 178
Aptamer 123
Argenio 165
Aurora 202
Autoimmune 197

B

Bahamondes 144
Bartlett 145
B-cell 104, 105, 182
Biological vii, 6, 18, 19, 99, 154, 194, 195
Biomarkers 159
Bonding 69
Boylan 46
Buccal 38, 39, 40, 41
Buffers 76
Burgess 203
Burlington 145

C

Cationic 98
Cavitation 113
Chapman 203
Chimeric 178
Choroid 111
Collagen 117, 118, 119
Consortium 181, 183
Cornea 110

D

Dekker 24, 25, 34, 46, 90, 144, 166, 202
Dendrimers 172, 191, 192
Density 69, 93
Dermis 49
Detergent 98
Diabetes 197, 198, 204
Dosage v, 2, 4, 24, 34, 69, 109, 125, 151
Droplet 78
Durasert 120

E

Edward 145
Emulsion 103
Enteric 33, 188
Enzymatic 75
Episcleral 119
Estrogen 131
Eugene 204
Exhalation 158
Expensive 28
Exposure 193
Extrusion 135

F

Farhan 108
Farokhzad 181, 182, 183
Fibrin 107
Fibroids 139
Follicular 131
Fusion 100

G

Gastric 65, 152
Gastro v, 63, 70
Gibaldi 24, 166

H

Hadgraft 145, 166
Handbook 24, 25, 166
Hepatic 74, 156, 158
Hormonal 106, 128, 129, 133, 134, 138
Humectants 77
Hybrid 174
Hydrogels 181, 191, 192, 207
Hypodermis 49

I

Inhalation 99, 152, 190
Inorganic 191
Insertion 113, 127
Insoluble 22, 115
Insulin 196, 197, 203
Intrinsic 9, 19
Inverse 93

K

Kaunitz 144
Kearns 166
Kinetics 135, 137, 154, 175
Kluwer 146

L

Langer 166, 181, 182, 203
Lieberman 108
Ligands 94, 195
Lippincott 166
Luteal 131

M

Mansour 144
Margalit 182
Mathiowitz 46
Membrane 43, 59, 75, 163
Menstrual 129, 131

Metabolic 136, 149, 204
Micelles 171, 191, 192
Mirena 145
Monoclonal vi, 104, 105, 106, 107, 108, 197, 203
Mucosa 46
Muller 112
Myocardial 107
Myometrium 129
Myosin 107

N

Nebulizer 83, 84
Niosomal 100
Niosome 101

O

Ocufit 117, 118
Ocusert 115, 119
Ointment 119
Ophthalmic 116
Opsonins 101
Oregon 204
Osmotic 24, 89, 90, 115, 163
Ovulation 131
Oxidation 187

P

Papillary 49
Parenteral 152, 189
Patches 189
Peipert 147
Peppas 166, 182
Peptide vii, 185, 187, 190, 192, 193, 196, 197, 198, 199, 200, 201, 204, 205
Peripheral 107
Permeation 42, 48, 51, 53, 57, 59
Pharmacy xi, 34, 108, 203
Plasma 4
Polyester 58

Polymeric 12, 90, 102, 134, 166, 171, 181, 191
Polyvinyl 57
Pregnancy 106
Prodrug 153
Prolong 35
Prostate 106
Pulmonary vi, 73, 78, 79, 85, 152, 158, 190

R

Rathbone 46, 145, 146, 166
Reprod 144, 145
Retention 114
Retina 111
Ribozyme 124
Ritschel 166, 202
Rowland 146, 166

S

Saliva 38, 43
Salivary 43
Scaffolds 174
Schumitzky 165
Sclera 111
Shanafelt 203
Sibalis 205
Sodium 76
Springer 146, 165, 205
Steril 145, 147
Swarbrick 46

T

Tahami 205
Torchilin 183, 204, 205

U

Uterine 139
Uterus 129, 132

V

Varghese 34, 108
Vesicles 99
Viscosity 76, 78, 93

W

Wilkins 166
Williams 166, 183
Wolters 146

Y

Yakugaku 206
Yamaguchi 204
Yanagi 206
Ycetal 203

Z

Zasshi 206

www.ingramcontent.com/pod-product-compliance
Lightning Source LLC
LaVergne TN
LVHW020425070526
838199LV00003B/285